P9-BBV-490

JAMES SCHALLER, M.D.

The Diagnosis and Treatment of

Babesia

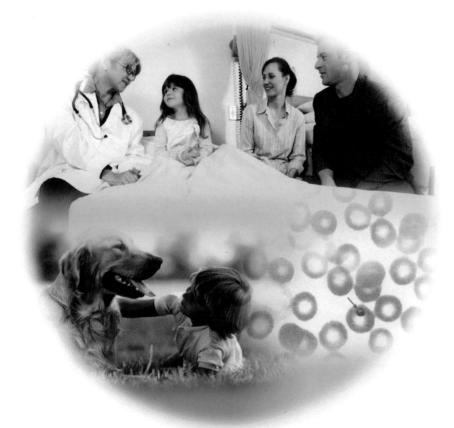

A Stealth Infection Routinely Ignored in American Medicine

Cover Art: Phil Chow
Illustrations: Jamie Joyce
Copy Editor: PJ Langhoff
Book Production: PJ Langhoff and Ronald Gombach
Research Assistant: Randall Blackwell

Hope Academic Press
Tampa, Florida

www.HopeAcademic.com

This book was partially supported by an unrestricted grant from the antibiotic specialty company QMEDRX.
www.QMedRx.com

To My Precious Son Jeremy,
Who Battled Babesia and Won!

And to Patients Naively Called "Crazy."

Acknowledgements

To Dr. Joseph Jemsek, Dr. Joe Burrascano,
Dr. Stephen Phillips, Dr. Lesley Fein, Dr. Michael Cichon,
Dr. Brian Fallon, Dr. Charles Ray Jones, Dr. Ray Stricker,
Dr. Alan MacDonald, Dr. Richard Horowitz, and
Ginger Savely NP, for helping thousands of patients with
advanced medical care decades ahead of your peers.
Your great sacrifice has saved many lives.

Lorraine Johnson, Esq. for caring for master healers as an
attorney's attorney. You are the cream of your guild.

To Pat Smith of the Lyme Disease Association for
giving away her life through service to so many victims of
severe Tick-borne infections throughout the United States.

You are my treasured heroes.

Informed Consent Disclaimer

Table of Contents

Individual Babesia Treatments in Detail

**Artemisinin's Amazing Ability to Kill
Red Blood Infections and Cancer**

❧

Babesia Symptoms and Signs

High fevers

Decreased appetite

Cough

Fatigue

Air hunger

Chills

Listlessness

Enlarged liver
(under your right rib cage)

Sweats

Muscle aches

Joint aches

Malaise

Headache

Depression

Jaundice (Yellow hue
on eyes, hands and skin)

Vomiting

Shortness of breath

Anxiety/Panic

Enlarged spleen
(under your left rib cage)

Nausea

Dark urine

Enlarged lymph nodes
(also in Lyme or Bartonella)

Why Study Babesia?

I grew up very close to my grandmother. Her firstborn son died and I was her first grandchild. So when I arrived, she became another mother, a best friend, a safe place, and a fan that cheered me to a master's degree and doctorate. In my grandmother's eyes, I could have been a street person, and still she would have loved me just as much. We talked many times about the loss of her son. He died from a hole in his heart, which is a defect that most cardiac surgeons can now easily fix.

The story of Babesia touches me as profoundly as did the earlier loss my grandmother suffered due to her son's heart defect. My own precious son was found to be suffering from Babesia, a serious, but little known and often overlooked infection bearing devastating consequences. Many physicians failed to notice my son was not "fine" and dismissed his eccentric dark eyes, excess fatigue and occasional fevers. A few tried to suggest that he was merely depressed. They did not grasp the idea that my son, who was so full of life, now had lost so much energy he could not act on any of his dreams, or even function from day-to-day.

As a physician who publishes in many areas of medicine, I was stunned to listen to so-called "experts" in infectious disease medicine who would offer sincere, but unreasonable diagnoses. So many smart physicians seemed cognitively frozen and rigid in their beliefs. Because of high patient volume, it would seem that many invest precious little time researching new medical practices and emergent diseases. As a result, these physicians are often limited in current practical knowledge due to the time constraints brought about by their hectic daily schedules.

Some physicians only understand Babesia when they have serious tick-based infections experienced by members of their own family. Sadly, even with an infected relative, recognition is not as common as one might think, or even hope.

Why do sincere physicians fail to see what is so plainly before them? Indeed, often they themselves are infected, their own insight is gone, and that is often the first thing lost in someone with a tick-borne infection. Yes, the physicians themselves are infected. It amazes me that in speaking with different physicians, I can easily see very subtle cognitive, character and personality changes – clear indicators of tick-borne illness. Unfortunately for them, I have to count them as lost, as most are too far gone to even hear me. I try to explain the facts of their illness to them, but they remain unreceptive despite the many pages of well-researched evidence presented to them.

Another compelling reason for me to write about Babesia is because of my love and respect for my patients. I oppose human pain in any of my patients. In this regard, Babesia is like chronic pain. The DEA, state medical boards and some

District Attorneys promote chronic pain by blatantly terrorizing pain experts.

In stark contrast to these practices, I have written this book in order to help end the pain and suffering caused by Babesia. I have seen effective cures for this illness and it is my goal to achieve this for you. Within the pages of this book I will teach you clinically important facts about this illness and all the major treatment options currently available. Most experts are in agreement that Babesia can be successfully treated. While doctors have different methods of treating Babesia, you should expect nothing less than a complete cure.

⚬⚬⚬

Joan came to see me after being treated for Lyme disease. She was from Orlando, Florida where Lyme disease is not supposed to exist, according to some "experts," because "no deer live in Florida." (A million deer live in Florida). Nevertheless, she did not ignore a uniform 4-inch rash she discovered following a recent camping trip in central Florida, which was initially diagnosed by a dermatologist as ring worm. Finally a nurse practitioner thought she might have Lyme, and treated her for 30 days. Joan thought that was going to be the end of it. But despite her nurse's comments that she "had been treated fully and aggressively," residual and troubling symptoms remained.

Over the next few years she slowly lost her ability to work due to fatigue and headaches. Because she lost her job, she found herself without any insurance. Then after several years, she was diagnosed with Babesia. Only after her diagnosis was she treated fully, and could return to work, fully recovered. Because her health care providers failed to diagnose her medical condition, she was handed a sentence of many lost years inside a medical prison.

Some Lyme experts feel that failing to diagnose Babesia is a very serious and dangerous mistake. And yet very few physicians, including infectious disease doctors, routinely check for Babesia, even though many studies show the infection exists in ticks all over the United States, and indeed throughout the world. If you are one of the few patients who have actually been diagnosed with Lyme and your concerns about possible Babesia have not been ignored or dismissed, then consider yourself blessed. In reality, even the smartest physicians will miss Babesia – it is not part of the American medical community's diagnostic alphabet.

Tick-Borne Illness: Knowing More Than God

I recently listened to a pompous infectious disease expert summarize tick-borne illness as if she was discussing first grade math. As I listened to her standard infectious disease monologue, I thought about my loved ones who have suffered so severely from similarly dismissive, simple medicine. I thought of my entire family whose disease states were overlooked, causing them to lose precious years of productive lives due to the beliefs echoed by her and many other so-called "experts." To me, this physician was clearly exhibiting impaired insight into her own medical knowledge.

What she communicated was repetitious, confusing and fil-tered quotes. She championed two flawed studies with a cer-tainty that was both verbally colorless and clinically danger-ous. If you were her patient and did not fit into the confines of this rigid study, then she would have no choice but to com-pletely ignore your illness. In my opinion there is no excuse for cult-like fanaticism that would place the value of power and prestige above human beings.

Having said this, let's begin our discussion with the basics of Babesia. Within the collective world, there are approximately 850 species of ticks.[1]

The kinds of infections that these ticks carry are both highly diverse and numerous. A single tick may carry any combina-tion of hundreds of different types of infections. Once inside the human body, some of these infections have the ability to alter their physical form in over twenty ways in order to evade the human immune system. If you are starting to feel like this is more than what you anticipated to learn, then welcome to the world of tick-borne illness.

In the last 30 years medical science has only begun to learn about just **one type** of tick-borne illness, Lyme disease. Despite all that has been learned to date, results utilizing even the crudest reporting methods indicate huge increases of tick-borne infection spreading throughout North America.

Museums display examples of ticks that contain Lyme, so we know that Lyme disease has been around for over a century, but we are only beginning to understand the complex nature of tick-borne infections. Indeed, it was a housewife and artist named Polly Murray who was responsible for discovering clinical American Lyme disease. She noted a flood of ill children living within her area whose illnesses had been missed by many New England medical centers. Initially, Lyme disease was seen simply as a form of arthritis. Misdiagnosing Lyme is a serious error on the physician's part, since Lyme bacteria migrate to the brain within days, and can also impact any human organ, and cause any of hundreds of possible symptoms. In reality, only 25% of Lyme patients with acute infection have arthritis.[2] Most Lyme patients present with a cluster of symptoms that defies simple explanation by any diagnostic "cookbook."

Any viewpoint which limits Lyme disease to the mere label of "Lyme arthritis," serves to limit your understanding of what is essentially a serious, systemic disease affecting the entire body.[3-5] The acceptance of this arthritis label by any member of the medical establishment shows the simplistic thinking still present. It shows we are struggling to master and define even one tick-borne infection – the most common tick illness in the United States.

Before we examine Babesia more closely, one should know that despite decades of research on Lyme disease, there still remains no reliable and universally agreed upon lab test designed to clearly detect all of the 100^+ Lyme strains found in the Americas and throughout the world. The accuracy of Lyme lab testing kits varies profoundly, and **some Lyme lab tests use Lyme strains or species that are not indigenous to the location of the patient who is being tested, and that is crucial to detecting their Lyme infection.**

The most commonly used Lyme test, called an ELISA test, consists of grinding up whole Lyme bacteria so that **huge amounts of junk particles are present within the testing medium.**[6,7] These particles can actually prevent or negate a true positive test result because our immune system reacts only with a very limited number of specific Lyme parts. With this in mind, is it any wonder that ELISA tests are often negative in patients who present with bulls-eye rashes—even many months after the initial Lyme rash appears, and when the body should have made plenty of Lyme antibodies? Or is it any surprise that licensed laboratories often return conflicting results for the same patient, with one test reading positive and another lab showing a negative result?[8,9]

As a physician myself, I am stunned that some physicians

would consider a junk test like an ELISA as a "credible screening test," when it returns false results in as much as 75% of those tested.[10,11]

Another crucial Lyme test, the Western Blot, is no longer generally useful because most labs have removed crucial Lyme proteins. So blood samples filled with antibodies against Lyme will not find Lyme proteins to bind in the test kit. You see, years ago, some labs were getting more positives then lab staff thought "reasonable," so they dummied down the test, causing many cases of Lyme to be missed. This happened in many of my family members including my children who did not meet CDC Lyme research criteria on Western Blots done at large national labs, when it was blatantly obvious they had Lyme. So the current ELISA and Western Blot Lyme testing done by most labs is grossly unreliable—like bobbing for apples without your teeth.

The question of inaccuracies in Lyme laboratory testing pales in comparison to Babesia, which is also an infection carried by ticks. We call Babesia a "co-infection" which rides tandem with Lyme, because as a trend in the United States, if you are infected with Babesia, you more than likely are carrying both of these infections.

Research scientists are just beginning to learn that substantially more Babesia exists than is currently recognized in the medical community. New species of Babesia are being discovered as I write, and those species are not weak, mildly symptomatic ones, causing something mild like a brief cold. We are finding new forms that cause severe illness and even death to humans living in the United States. These new strains are being discovered by virtue of the intense symptoms and strength of illness they cause, much like a volcano is "discovered" because no one can ignore ten miles of explosive ash.

Further, we are finding aggressive new strains of Babesia in some of our most heavily populated states, including regions with respected medical research centers, but which fail to find these infections. With the surging tide of Babesia charging forward, we are faced with the reality of our limited knowledge about this disease. More specifically, very little information exists in commonly researched medical sites like *PubMed*, a site which catalogues 16 million articles. Only a few years ago, less than 50 references on Lyme and co-infections were cited in *PubMed*.

This deficit in detailed information about Babesia makes the current scanty information on extremely rare forms of cancer seem like a literary surplus. In general, speaking with medical certainty or authority about Babesia infections in humans during this time of basic discovery, would show an "expert" individual lacked both good judgment and a sense of sobriety.[12]

Human Babesia is Not a Rare Find

For clinicians, researchers, professional expert witnesses and state board appointees, it is time to be humble, and realize we are just beginning our journey into tick-borne diseases, a discovery process that will very likely be decades in length.

Babesia expert Dr. Gutierrez suggests that after examining Babesia studies from many areas around the world, **Babesia could prove in fact to be a common infection, and not rare at all, as is currently thought.**[13] For example, he quotes Leeflang's work in which 54% of 173 Nigerian men were examined and whose blood proved to carry antibodies to Babesia.[14] Since physicians in Nigeria are routinely faced with another red blood cell parasite by the name of malaria, it is amazing they would ever take note of Babesia at all.

Another study done in the 1970's shows that Mexico, right off of our border, had Babesia infections in approximately 36% of people who were tested. Among those tested, research indicated the subjects were not reacting with the expected antibodies to the most common United States Babesia, which is the species *microti*, but instead to Babesia *canis*, a type of Babesia that more commonly infects dogs than their human counterparts.[15]

We do not know how many patients in the United States currently harbor the illness Babesia. An assumption that the numbers are only a few dozen per state is probably a birthday wish. Physician apathy about Babesia is apparent when we are already aware that **3-8% of blood donors have Babesia microti.** Indeed, in some western coastal states, antibodies against some type of Babesia-like organism may already be present at a rate of 15% of the population.[16]

Possible Signs and Symptoms of Babesia

Symptoms in Babesia-Infected Cattle

Babesia infected cattle offer some lessons for humankind. Once infected by this virulent organism, these animals develop the following signs and symptoms:

- High fever

- Malaise

- Listlessness

- Decreased appetite

- Reduced weight

- Red urine

- Anemia

- Jaundice or a yellowing of the eyes and skin

- Internal organ damage

Symptoms of Babesia Infection in Humans

Babesia can cause serious symptoms, or virtually no symptoms at all. Some of Babesia's more serious symptoms are the cause of confusing and unexplainable lab results and curious biopsies. When infected, some people immediately have a fever and fatigue, while other people do not become ill for years. Every person and their disease process is absolutely unique in nature.

Some well-meaning physicians will tell their patients that they are cured because their "objective" symptoms and signs are gone. I have met many so-called "cured" patients who came to me after visiting academic medical centers. This definition of "cure" is rather shortsighted. While it is true the patient may no longer feel feverish or dehydrated, they can hardly be considered cured. Unfortunately for the patients, some clinicians will attempt to dismiss their patient's subtle residual symptoms as "subjective." Their dangerously complacent definition means that the patient's symptoms are merely *something they are complaining about*, which invalidates both the patient's knowledge of their own body, as well as their existing disease.

Another diagnostic problem among Babesia victims is that they will not usually report being bitten by a deer tick or other possible infectious agent. Deer ticks are stealthy and in their larval state, can be as small as poppy seeds. At the time of the bite, they inject painkillers, antihistamines and anticoagulants that allow them to go virtually undetected.[17]

Any amount of time spent outdoors in any suburb or country setting is worth noting. Many patients will minimize the fact that they spent a **few hours** camping, hiking, hunting, nature walking, and inland boating. It is important to note possible tick exposure on any pets that have been outdoors as well. Additionally, contact with any outdoor animals, e.g., horses, can pass on a tick.

Here are examples of signs and symptoms of human infection from Babesia. Please note that some people with this infection have no symptoms. Please circle any symptom that may have applied to you within the last ten years:

- High fevers
- Slowed thinking
- Listlessness
- Decreased appetite
- Chills
- Sweats
- Headache
- Fatigue

- Muscle aches

- Joint aches/pain

- Depression

- Anxiety/Panic

- Nausea

- Vomiting

- Cough

- Shortness of breath

- Air hunger or unsatisfying deep breaths

- Dark urine

- Enlarged liver (under your right rib cage)

- Enlarged spleen (under your left rib cage)

- Yellow hue on eyes, hands and skin (Jaundice)

- Enlarged lymph nodes (also in Lyme or Bartonella)

- Significant memory change

- Profound psychiatric illnesses

- Struggle organizing

- Daytime sleep urgency despite nighttime sleep

- Waves of generalized itching

- Balance problems with dizziness

- Severe chest wall pains

- Random stabbing pains

- Weight loss

- Sensitivity to light

- Sleep in excess of 8 1/2 hours per day

- You have received blood from another person

Some people are bitten by a very tiny deer tick, (no larger than the period at the end of this sentence). These ticks will not merely infect their victims with up to 100,000 Lyme spirochetes, but they will also infect them with Babesia at the same time. Some clinicians feel that if you experience a *sudden high fever, sweats and chills* within the first two weeks following a bite, or even periodically thereafter, you should seriously consider Babesia as the culprit, and not assume the symptoms are from Lyme disease. If you do become infected with Babesia, you should know that it immediately enters your red blood cells. Studies offer different ratios concerning Lyme disease and various co-infections. The range of Lyme patients who are also infected with Babesia is reported to be approximately 12%-66%.

Frankly, we do not know how many people with Lyme also have Babesia, because we have no idea how many Americans have undiagnosed Lyme disease. In one study, only 1 in 40 Lyme patients were shown to have been reported to their regional health department, despite state-level mandatory reporting requirements for Lyme disease. Furthermore, these patients typically visited clinicians who utilized labs that were not equipped to properly detect Lyme disease.

What to Expect if You Have Both Lyme and Babesia

When both infections are present, the initial signs and symptoms can often be exactly the same, but are usually reported as significantly more intense, severe and longer lasting. Lyme and Babesia attack the body differently, and most clinicians agree that treating patients with both infections is significantly more difficult.

One reason that treating both infections simultaneously is challenging is that most Babesia treatments target red blood cell infections in the same manner as malaria. The drugs utilized to treat Babesia are **not** the same treatments used to treat Lyme disease. Babesia treatments attempt to kill red blood cell parasites, while Lyme disease treatments work to kill Lyme bacteria.

The following are key summary observations of Babesia microti:

• Human Babesiosis (Babesia infection) can apparently be a silent infection.

• When untreated, a silent Babesial infection may persist for many years.

• Silent infections are found in about one-third of infected people, and that status may change into an active infection at any time.

• While Babesia can sometimes be **initially detected** in the blood samples of infected patients, more typically no Babesia can be visualized using routine blood smears as soon as a week after the onset of illness.

• When patients had blood-borne DNA positive for Babesia, they also had persistent symptoms of Babesiosis.

• As a trend, if antibodies against Babesia were detected at high levels, Babesial DNA was more likely to be found.

• Physicians tend not to recognize Babesial infection in those who are concurrently infected with Lyme disease, because Babesia symptoms tend to mimic those caused by Lyme disease.

• Patients with moderate to severe Lyme disease should obtain diagnostic tests for Babesiosis and possibly other tick-borne pathogens, especially in patients having a delayed or poor response to antibiotic treatment.[18]

- The presence of Babesia seems to weaken the ability of the body to fight Lyme disease. For example, Lyme DNA was more often detected and remained within the blood longer when a patient was also infected with Babesia.

- Babesial infections can impair human defenses, which will then allow Lyme to be more aggressive in causing symptoms in the joints, heart, peripheral nerves and brain.

- Whenever someone is diagnosed with "moderate to severe Lyme Disease," Babesia should always be considered as a possible co-infection.[19,20]

Babesia as a Mild Illness

I once had a patient whose blood testing for Babesia was sent to a "junk" lab. A junk lab may be defined as a laboratory that is ill-equipped by either experience or technology to process lab tests accurately. This lab could not diagnosis a tick infection if it had been physically crawling out of the blood sample. The patient lived in a hyper-epidemic area, and as luck would have it, the test returned as positive. The patient was a hard worker, and yet he had been frustrated that he had to drink **ten cups of coffee per day** just to keep himself awake.

I made the mistake of thinking that his family doctor was knowledgeable on the topic of Babesia, and asked him to treat the man. The doctor informed his patient that he could not have Babesia, because he would be deathly ill if he did have it. Unfortunately for his patient, this physician had not read even the basic information that appears in most medical text-books – many patients with Babesia (microti) living in the United States **do not have symptoms.** The Babesia forms found in countries like Europe do seem to cause more severe illness, but many infected people in America have no symptoms at all, or at least initially.

Babesia — the Deadly Stealth Illness

We really do not know how many children and adults die each year from Babesia. Many researchers place the fatality rate at approximately 5%, yet much Babesia microti escapes detection and other forms of the parasite are unfamiliar to most physicians. Newer forms such as Babesia *duncani* are dangerous and routinely missed.

According to Babesia expert Patricia Conrad, Professor of Veterinary Medicine at the University of California, some human cases of Babesia are being completely ignored. As a treating physician, I agree. When I ask research microbiologists and infection researchers about Babesia, if they look at me with glossy eyes, I know that my patients are in trouble. **The medical establishment cannot see, diagnosis or treat what it does not know, or will not acknowledge.**

The danger with some forms of American Babesia is that patients with symptoms or health problems severe enough to send them to the local emergency room are presenting with an illness that no one is qualified to diagnose.

Our Babesia understanding is so poor that we are still discovering new species producing significant illness in humans, like Babesia duncani.[21] This new strain does not harm humans in the manner in which a physician might expect, which would be by exploding red blood cells. For example, Dr. Conrad explained how Babesia duncani-infected hamsters died by **fluid filling their lungs.** The same thing can happen in infected humans. These lung symptoms and others are routinely missed in ER's.

This year, many adults and children will go to an emergency room or their family physician for the following serious symptoms:

- Shortness of breath
- Unusual swelling
- Fatigue
- Poor appetite
- Intermittent fever
- Headache
- Chills

- Nausea/vomiting

- Emotional liability

- An unproductive cough

- A sore throat

- Light sensitivity

- Belly pain

- Weakness

- Menopause or perimenopause

- "Old age"

- Poor long-term functioning

Dr. Conrad and I are both concerned that these symptoms are overlooked signs of Babesia. We believe some Babesia infections are routinely diagnosed as basic asthma, a psychiatric diagnosis, or even sweating from perimenopause or flu. One way that Babesia escapes detection by your family doctor or emergency room physician is that **it does not cause anemia** – your red blood cell number is normal, so you are sent home. You are discharged because your breathing or temperature returns to normal, and the true cause of the illness is entirely missed – Babesia. In one animal study, a horse died of severe shortness of breath and fluid in the lungs.[22] This reminds me of a case where two people with Babesia had **no signs of anemia in their blood**. But a Babesia expert told their doctors to check for the presence of **microscopic signs of broken blood cells** in their urine samples and they eventually found their patients positive for hemoglobin. Both patients had Babesia, and their illnesses had been missed by many intelligent physicians.[23]

What Happens When Doctors Miss <u>Active</u> Babesia?

You or your loved one can die or become dangerously ill from a wide range of serious Babesia symptoms such as:

- Heart attacks
- Heart failure
- Severe fatal low blood pressure
- Shock
- Respiratory distress with poor oxygenation of the blood
- Kidney failure
- Diffuse full body bleeding[24]

To prevent these negative outcomes, physicians should learn that **unexplained fever, shortness of breath, or both should raise suspicions of Babesia.** When considering this infection, physicians need to order a CBC or blood smear to be performed "manually." What is a manual examination of blood? It involves a real laboratory expert searching under a very high-powered microscope to find Babesia. The organism will appear as tiny infections inside the red blood cells. This infection is not easy to see, especially if the blood exam is rushed, or the wrong stain or the wrong technique is used.

In our highly technical world, we might think a blood examination by a machine would be less prone to tired eyes, distractions, and error. In fact, machines that examine blood are extremely poor at recognizing Babesia inside red blood cells, and a machine evaluation offers false confidence that Babesia is not present.

Physicians and Babesia: A Summary

- **Most physicians wrongly believe that the flu is just the flu and never consider Babesia when a significant fever presents.**

- **Virtually no physician thinks to order testing for Babesia.**

- **No Babesia training is offered during medical school or residency.**

- **Physicians cannot diagnose what they do not think exists.**

- **Most physicians do not realize that Babesia can kill people.**

When I examined a case where a child died from a new strain of Babesia, it is clear from the account of the baby's care, that the physicians tried everything they could possibly think of to save the child. Unfortunately however, Babesia was never even considered. The time has come for clinicians to consider

Babesia in any patient presenting with the signs and symptoms mentioned previously.[25]

Babesia Denial vs. Malaria: Repeating Past History

As one Nobel prize winner once reported, "The agent of malaria did not resemble bacteria, and was present in strange forms, and...it was completely outside the circle of the known pathogenic microbes, and many observers, not knowing how to classify it, found it simpler to doubt its existence."[26]

Presently 200 to 500 million people all over the world become infected with malaria each year. With numbers of that size, how can we ignore or miss another malaria-like infection that sits like a massive elephant in the center of the medical waiting room?

Medicine has always been blessed with clinicians of visionary creativity. Conservative physicians initially horribly abused these brilliant men and women. For example, George Washington was dying and was told that he needed to be treated with leeches according to the academic doctors of the time, but a smart, creative doctor told him he needed a tracheotomy to breathe. Of course the latter was correct and Washington survived.[27]

Similarly, a small group of clinically alert physicians know that Babesia is not a rare infection. These doctors are the few who are saving many lives. They know that Babesia is present in many more folks then just a few patients with HIV or absent spleens. (The spleen's function is to clean the blood of parasites).

Another way American medicine ignores Babesia is by failing to report cases of it. Dr. Sherr is often asked to treat very ill patients, and some of these individuals have Babesia. When she tries to report her findings to the state Health Department, they dismiss her claims and have actually told her, "Ignore the diagnosis of babesiosis because it is just **trendy**. It is not a medical problem in Pennsylvania." I suppose that to them, it would only become a "real" problem if they or their loved ones would have it.[28,29,30]

Babesia Causes Significant Fatigue

While it may be "trendy" to be terribly tired, Kevin did not think so. He worked as an investment planner and enjoyed doing his own yard work in Texas. One week he thought he had a cold that grew bad enough that he took off three days from work. His fever was 102.4. He successfully treated his fever with repeated doses of 1500 mg of Tylenol. His physician then gave him a "Z-PAK" of Zithromax, (five tablets at 250mg strength). When he was still slightly ill, his family doctor referred him to an infectious disease expert. The infectious disease physician tested a couple tubes of his blood, and diagnosed "a very aggressive flu." Kevin's doctor said, "The fact that your temperature is already within a normal range is a good sign."

Nine months later Kevin was fired. He believed it was caused by difficulty getting to work on time and also daytime fatigue. Some of his friends at work asked him if he was drinking or taking sedatives. He drank five cups of coffee a day and smoked three packs of stimulating nicotine-filled cigarettes each day, but was still too tired to work at his previous energy levels.

His wife eventually sought a marital separation because she could not handle his "problems" any more. She left with their two children and moved back to her parent's home in another state.

Then Keven went to four other physicians and was diagnosed with fibromyalgia, chronic fatigue syndrome, and a sleep disorder. A sleep study showed some restless leg movement, but the medical treatment of a low dose of Klonopin, had no apparent benefit.

Kevin was eventually diagnosed with Babesia and Lyme disease, and after an extended period of treatment for each infection, he is now working successfully and has reconciled with his wife.

Babesia Symptoms are Diverse

Babesia causes symptoms from past injuries to worsen. An old sports injury might suddenly hurt more. Headaches may trouble you and medication may or may not help the headache. Babesia weakens the body's immune system so that the Lyme spirochetes can increase in number. Lyme may further undermine your personality, thinking processes, joint health, mood, balance and heart health.[31]

Lyme and Babesia: Why Treatments Fail

Throughout this book we will be explaining why you might not be experiencing a full recovery following treatment. Some exhausted patients are not getting healthy because of residual Lyme and Babesia and other related reasons. Below are common reasons for treatment failure.

1) The antibiotic treatment is not aggressive enough, and the dose needs to be increased.

2) Treatment length was too short, causing a Babesia or Lyme relapse. Babesia or Lyme is not cured with one simple antibiotic, prescribed universally at the same dosages and identical treatment durations.

3) Babesia was treated only once. Much malaria research shows that malaria is a "smart" bug and that it learns how to evade a single treatment. This process may also apply to the Babesia organism.

4) The medication is simply a poor fit to kill Babesia and a different one would be more effective.

5) You have other co-infections along with Babesia. For example, perhaps you have a very aggressive form of Bartonella, another tick-borne infection, which is common and causes many medical and emotional symptoms such as anger, panic, irritability, rage, anxiety, and OCD.

6) You are exposed to one of the 30% of US buildings harboring indoor mold biotoxins. Any structure having unresolved leaks that are not repaired within two days or which has humidity routinely above 65% might have excessive mold behind walls, ceilings, baseboards or residing in the air ducts.

7) You are unable to remove Lyme or mold biotoxins from your body. This capability can be determined by getting a full five-part HLA DRB, DQB test done by LabCorp (Test code number 012542). This test will show you your genetic pattern, and this will show how good you are at removing these biotoxins. If you have the 16-5-51 or 15-6-51 pattern you will not remove Lyme's outer toxins without taking a special binder. These Lyme biotoxins are very powerful and are not passive. They are able to disrupt and under-

mine many systems in the human body. Therefore, administering aggressive antibiotics in this subgroup actually makes them profoundly chronically ill, and can cause serious body harm, e.g. dropping anti-inflammation hormones and proteins to uselessly low levels in weeks, and causing diffuse types of autoimmunity.

8) The treatment is too aggressive. The antibiotics alone or the antibiotics plus Babesia/Lyme die-off is too rapid, causing restlessness, painful joints, headaches, trouble thinking, fatigue and other ill feelings.

Babesia Requires Special Treatment

It is critical to realize that Babesia is **not** a bacteria like Lyme disease. So the treatments used for Lyme typically do not work on the Babesia organism. You do not saw a piece of wood with a wrench—meaning the medications used to treat Babesia are usually malaria medications. Babesia is loosely related to malaria. Both are parasites that live within the red blood cells. So the idea that a broad-spectrum antibiotic will remove Babesia is actually a false conclusion.

A Simple Explanation of Babesia Infection

The most common carrier of Babesia is a virtually invisible larval deer tick. One state trooper who has been bitten many times while in the Carolinas told me that he has never seen a deer tick. Unfortunately for him, his labs clearly showed otherwise.

Babesia-Fueled Animal Plagues

We have learned a great deal about human Babesia by studying how Babesia attacks animals.

Babesia has been around a long time and researchers think it might have been the cause of the Biblical plague against livestock described in the Bible's *Exodus*.[32] We do know that Babesia is generally carried and spread by ticks. In the United States, while Babesia-caused human infections are currently carried by very tiny deer ticks, in the 1890's another type of tick carried Babesia *bigemina* and caused massive illness to cattle in the southeastern states. This type of illness was called "Texas fever," or "Texas red water fever." At the time, it killed 50% of the infected cattle in the United States, while similarly Australia lost millions of cows to this Babesia infection. Many cows died within a week of exhibiting serious symptoms. How long the animals had the infection before becoming ill is still unknown.[33]

This cattle-loving tick has been obliterated from the United States, but it exists elsewhere in the world. They were removed from the US by tick-control methods like dipping the cattle in a tick-killing agent, inoculating young cattle with a mild and weakened form of Babesia to stimulate their immune systems, and limiting the movement of northern herds of cattle that would have moved south. The result of these various control measures was nothing short of amazing. In contrast to human Babesia, this fatal form of animal Babesia was completely erased from the US map. The tick that carried this Babesia bigemina infection no longer exists in the United States.

The medicines used in these cattle may help us in human treatment methods. Some Babesia medications were strong enough for the animals to recover completely, while other Babesia medications removed the signs and symptoms yet still allowed residual amounts of Babesia to remain in the animals' bodies.[34]

Babesia in Recent Human History

Of the 100 different species of Babesia, the first suspected human Babesial infection was in 1908, and the first clearly reported human case was in 1957, diagnosed in a Yugoslavian cattle farmer. The first American case was reported in Nantucket, Massachusetts in 1969.[35] I suspect that Babesia is very similar to Lyme. We already know that Lyme disease can be found in museum specimens of ticks that are over a hundred years old. When new conditions existed that allowed for explosive growth (such as the complete removal of deer predators), Babesia became more common.[36] Babesia has increased largely due to the explosive deer population. Wild deer once hunted to near extinction, now overrun both suburbs and rural settings. Deer populations are so large that I actually have had a close friend who hit three deer with three different cars within an eight-week time period. The expansion of our human habitat of suburban lots peppered with scenic trees and brush has increased the population of various species of deer ticks and has resulted in an explosion of Babesia in the past several decades.

In the mid-1970's, physicians diagnosing Babesia in humans had to think of new treatments outside the routine FDA-approved guidelines. In fact, people were becoming ill with Babesia who had no exposure to livestock (which might carry divergens or bovis forms). Some patients had no clear exposure to rodents either, (which might carry microti form). Also, the range of B. microti was found to be far broader than a handful of New England states as was previously believed.

Research shows that Babesia is on the move and the tiny deer ticks that carry it are also aggressively entering virtually all parts of the United States. Further, many different types of animals such as skunks and raccoons have been found to carry forms of Babesia, so scientists and physicians are slowly becoming aware that Babesia is not limited to small New England towns. Even more surprising was the fact that some patients were becoming infected from blood transfusions from donations throughout the United States, including on the West Coast.[37-39]

A couple of years ago, an ill physician looked at her own blood under a very high-powered microscope. She found what she thought to be another unique species of Babesia. She showed it to infectious disease experts and pathologists. They were unable to identify it. I will discuss all the known forms of Babesia, including new forms, which can infect humans. As our highly basic understanding of human Babesia grows, we may indeed find additional species that can infect humans.

Treating Unidentified Forms of Babesia

A number of human Babesia forms currently exist which cannot be identified by most labs. Below, I list some samples of new Babesia types known to parasite research experts, but **unknown** to average clinical physicians. Why would this fact matter to you? If you miraculously convince a physician to test you for Babesia, you will still not easily be diagnosed. Why? **No routine human laboratory in the United States can diagnose the various forms of Babesia, period. And since physicians only acknowledge the results that labs present to them, your Babesia will be missed.**

Babesia Diagnosed Without Lab Testing

An expert in chronic Lyme disease was treating a man suffering from horrible migraines. This patient had previously failed to find a solution to his pain, even after consulting with neurologists and pain specialists at the Mayo Clinic, Yale, the Cleveland Clinic, and the University of Pennsylvania. He consulted with many smart, talented and reasonable physicians at these medical centers. They performed aggressive testing and exams but they could not find a reason for his pain except to tell him that he had "migraines."

My first question would be, "Why does this patient have headaches? What is causing the migraine?" The word "migraine" is not necessarily the ultimate illness–it might just be a banner symptom for a different illness. I routinely find that a wide range of tick infections can cause untreatable headaches. These tick infections directly or indirectly can cause low levels of anti-inflammation chemicals, such as MSH or VIP levels. So the levels of these pain-reducing hormones can fall due to various tick infections or from the biotoxins they create. These biotoxins then lower MSH and VIP, which are both super anti-inflammation chemicals that would have the ability to increase the body's natural narcotics. These important natural body chemicals are almost never tested.

The Lyme physician explained to this "migraine" patient that it was **"virtually impossible to completely rule out *all types* of Babesia."** This doctor added that since the man's headaches had failed to respond to literally 30-40 FDA approved treatments, treating a possibly "unidentified" Babesia might be a good idea. The man had no positive labs for Babesia microti or Babesia divergens. After five months of Babesia treatment, his terrible migraines that had lasted a total of thirteen years were completely gone. This man had no other obvious Babesia symptoms.

This man had testing done to look for the most common Babesia microti form. But even Babesia microti can be missed during testing. We must ask why that is. The microti may be present in only a small number of red blood cells, so tests that use only one drop of blood can easily miss its presence. Red blood cell testing commonly does not allow for a clear view of possible Babesia forms due to the need for oversized magnification, special stains and extended time looking under the microscope.

Deer Ticks are on the Move

I was recently told by an infectious disease physician that Babesia could not be in Pennsylvania or New York because as he put it, "deer ticks are largely limited to New England." I was so shocked by this statement that I could not speak.

Deer ticks are common and bite many individuals without their victim's awareness. For example, in a powerful study of San Francisco bay individuals, researchers were able to detect antibodies against the saliva of deer ticks in 36% of human blood samples tested. This means that 36% of these San Francisco bay residents had been bitten by deer ticks. This is the only way that so many people would have antibodies against deer tick saliva.[40]

Tick Identification Guide

Ixodes scapularis (includes deer tick)

Transmits agents of:
Lyme, babesiosis, Ehrlichiosis, Powassan encephalitis.

<u>Possibly transmits:</u> tick paralysis, tularemia, bartonella.

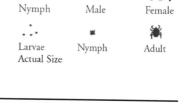

Amblyomma americanum (includes lone star tick)

Transmits agents of:
Ehrlichiosis, Lyme or Lyme-like illness, tularemia.

<u>Possibly transmits:</u> tick paralysis, Rocky Mt. spotted fever.

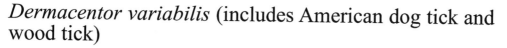

Dermacentor variabilis (includes American dog tick and wood tick)

<u>Transmits agents of:</u>
Rocky Mt. spotted fever, tularemia.

<u>Possibly transmits:</u> Ehrlichiosis. A small percentage of dog ticks carry the Lyme bacteria.

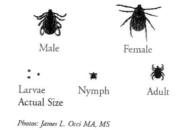

Photos: James L. Occi MA, MS

(Thanks to the Lyme Disease Association which makes the above images free on their web site at: http://www.lymediseaseassociation.org/Tickmark.pdf.)

Deer ticks carry both Lyme disease and Babesia. Their habitat is expanding all over the North American continent. They are found as southeast as the state of Florida (which has one million deer), to the northern Canadian provinces of Nova Scotia and Prince Edward Island, and west to the Dakotas, and southwest to Mexico. A small sample of states has published brief studies reporting deer ticks carrying Babesia. They have been found in Pennsylvania, New Jersey, Delaware, and the entirety of New England, Minnesota, Wisconsin, Maryland, North Carolina and Georgia.[41-48]

In the same manner that deer ticks are migrating by attaching to many mammals and birds, deer ticks infect migrating people. As a physician working in Florida, I routinely see individuals visiting for a few days or months states harboring huge deer tick populations, who then return to Florida infected. Of course, Florida brush and wilderness areas also have their own ticks, with perhaps the most commonly exposed patients being hunters, campers, nature walkers and those with deer living near their residences or workplace.

Deer ticks migrate by attachment to many creatures. They feed upon at least 125 species of North American vertebrates (54 mammals, 57 birds, and 14 lizard species), all migratory. Some of their favorite targets are white-tailed deer, cattle, dogs, a wide array of mice, small mammals and ground loving birds, which seem to help in deer tick dispersal.[49-52] On one occasion a pediatrician reported that one of his cured pediatric

Lyme patients was in New York City when a bird flew over him and dropped a deer tick onto his arm. Needless to say, the youth was not pleased with the event. While large cities may have low exposure risk to Lyme and Babesia, this extreme example shows how easily tick migration can be achieved.[53]

Deer Ticks and Babesia

While deer ticks are dispersing throughout the United States, some might wonder just how many are actually carrying Babesia.

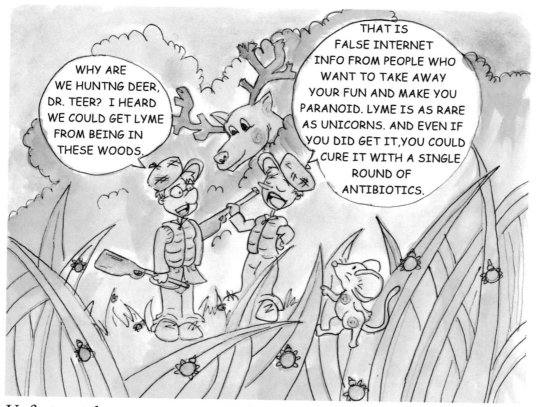

Unfortunately many smart and sincere people naively believe that the explosion of the United States deer population is trivial in terms of the risk for Lyme and Babesia infections. Their desire to offer kind reassurance ignores the reality of Lyme and Babesia's profound disbursal throughout America.

Twenty years ago a study showed that deer ticks were both plentiful and carried Babesia at approximately the same frequency as they carried Lyme. In this study it is amazing to read the number of infected ticks found *per hour* in a populated East Coast region.[54]

> **17** Babesia infected ticks **per hour per person**
> **16** Lyme infected ticks **per hour per person**

What is staggering to note is that these deer ticks carry **a little more Babesia than Lyme**. So the notion that Babesia is rare, is seriously flawed.[55]

High Babesia Infection Rates in Animals which Spread Babesia to Humans

In some areas of the United States, many animals that have deer ticks carry Babesia and therefore spread it to humans at a high level. For example, one sample regional area found that 80% of the mice that carried deer ticks were infected with Lyme, Babesia or Ehrlichia. 40% were infected with at least two of these infections. **In this context, the idea that Babesia is not a major health issue is simply a serious lack of education.**[56-59]

The End to Using Lyme as the Screening Infection

Many physicians with an expertise in tick infections became concerned when they noticed patients from all over the world carrying other tick infections but no Lyme infection. In the United States, most physicians think that if a person does not have a Lyme infection, it is likely they do not also have a co-infection. But this assumption is simply untrue. Patients can have any mix of tick-borne infections and that mix can exclude Lyme. **So interviewing, examining, and limiting lab testing to only one infection such as Lyme when a tick bite is suspected, is medical error.**

For example, in one study in the American Journal of Epidemiology, 19 people were diagnosed with erhlichia. Of those diagnosed, only one-third had Lyme and another third had Babesia.

So any physician who refuses to consider Babesia **only** after finding Lyme signs, symptoms and Lyme-positive lab test results, is offering only fair medical care. As one paper states, "In settings in which Lyme is found, **laboratory testing for co-infection is indicated (or should be done)** to ensure that appropriate antimicrobial treatment is given." In other words, **routinely ignoring possible Lyme co-infections is poor medical care.**[60]

This should come as no surprise since as early as twenty years ago, in areas with known Lyme and Babesia, **66% of Lyme patients also had Babesia.**[61] Further, in people with one tick-borne infection, up to 39% of these individuals had another tick infection. **The most commonly found co-infection with Lyme disease is Babesia.** In the Eastern United States, if a person has a co-infection, 80% of the time that infection is Babesia.[62-64]

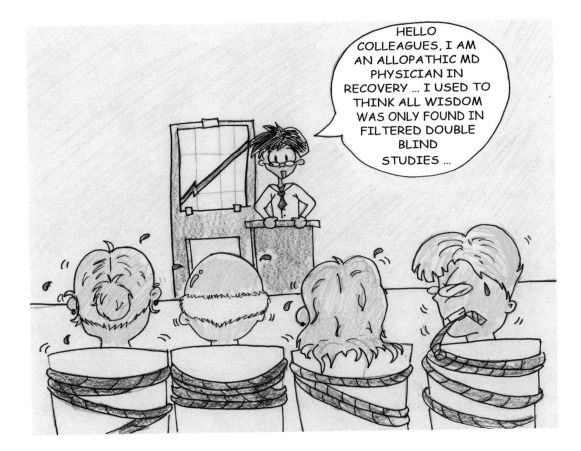

The clinical reality is it will be decades before all the forms of human Babesia are studied in double-blind studies.

How Many Annual Cases of Babesia are Diagnosed in the United States?

It took 50 years to diagnose just **one case** of human Babesia and another 50 years to discover some other dangerous American types that also infect humans. Common sense says we have hardly mastered this illness. Therefore, almost any physician who claims expertise about Babesia illness surely lacks significant knowledge.

For example, just today, thousands of people went to the emergency room with a high fever. Some were discharged with a fever of "unknown origin." An unknown percentage of these patients have Babesia. Any official-looking publication that will tell you that your state has had 20, 200, or 2,000 cases of Babesia this last year is guessing about Babesia detection. **We simply have no idea how many Americans have Babesia.**

Some physicians say, "Isn't Babesia an obscure tropical disease?" Their question indicates they do not have the ability to diagnose Babesia.

Babesia is not a bright glowing organism that dances across a microscope slide and waves to the pathologist. Babesia is extremely hard to see and requires advanced and repeated training. It has many unusual forms only recognizable under a microscope using special techniques. Since it is not a routine part of our surgery and pharmaceutical world, it is easier just to ignore its presence, considerate it immensely rare, and act as if it does not exist.

Amazingly, national health centers, Health Departments in states like Pennsylvania, and many local county Health Departments refuse to accept reported cases of Babesia for official registration. **Some agencies have actually asked not to be bothered.** So measuring a local epidemic is impossible.

Since approximately only 1 out of 40 physicians report **mandated** Lyme cases, and these "positives" are often diagnosed with poor labs, some believe we might be grossly underestimating the incidence of Lyme and Babesia. Indeed, Dr. Virginia Sherr's small study in the Pennsylvania suburbs, found 35 Babesia-positive patients by two CLIA-approved labs utilizing different technologies within only 14 months of time. These patients were tested from her modestly sized practice. **Imagine how many cases would be found if government agencies actually looked for Babesia instead of rejecting reports. Whatever the real frequency of Babesia, it is certainly not the low numbers published by some health departments and government agencies.**[65,66]

Diagnostic and Lab Problems

As virtual first-graders in Babesia medicine, we are making many mistakes. For example, in the 1970's, some thought that Babesia was the *cause* of the Lyme outbreaks in New England, as some ill patients were found to also be positive for

Babesia microti in these new Lyme endemic areas. Eventually it was clarified that Babesia was common, but not the *cause* of Lyme. Then it seemed that for New England physicians, Babesia suddenly fell off the map.

Another example of our limited Babesia understanding is a simple comparison of our Babesia research from 2000 as compared to 2006. Species believed to exist only in Europe or solely in animals, are now being reported in humans in the United States. New human Babesia infections are being discovered all the time.[67-69] A respected book published in 2000 reported only four types of human Babesia (B):

B. microti

B. divergens

B. bovis

B. equi[70]

Some physicians are not even aware of these four species and think that the only form of Babesia in the United States is Babesia microti. Few labs in the U.S. can test for any form other than B. microti. And while B. microti is probably the most common form in the United States, pathologist Dr. Alan MacDonald was finding **non**-microti Babesia in New York during the 1980's. Those strains were proven to be living Babesia forms. This was done by inserting the infected blood cells into hamsters which would subsequently develop classic signs of Babesia red blood cell infection.

Here we are in 2006, and we are still finding new dangerous forms. **Perhaps the only reason we know new ones exist is because when they do occur, they produce significant illness and are occasionally deadly,** making them impossible to ignore. We do not know how many other Babesia species exist in the United States, especially examples that are missed because they only cause modest illness.

Below is a list of the currently recognized forms of human Babesia found in America. In the first example, WA1-3 represents a form of Babesia first found in Washington State (WA) and the three patients who first had this unique form of Babesia are numbered 1-3. Another form is called CA1-4, which means this was initially identified in California (CA) and four people (1-4) have been identified with this unique infection.

Forms that can Infect Humans as of 2006:

WA1-3: Three patients with this unique Washington state (WA) form.[71-76]

CA1-4: Four patients with unique California (CA) form.[77]

CA5,6: Two more California patients with a unique Babesia.[78]

B. duncani: A new species that includes both WA1-3, and CA5,6 and can be either mild or aggressive. This is a very serious discovery because this form does not appear to be rare. For example, one of the first patients found with this species of Babesia (WA1), had neighbors with high antibodies showing infection with WA1. How rare could this be if four folks on the same street are positive? Further, WA-1 has increasingly been found in the western states, including California, the most populated state in the US. The symptoms of these patients range from no signs of illness, to a mild infection or "flu," to severe illness.[79-84]

MO1: Discovered in a Missouri patient, so it is identified as MO.[85]

B. odocoilei: A type of Babesia found in select deer but which can also infect humans.[86-90]

EU1: A form discovered in Europe and abbreviated EU. However, over time, Babesia forms which are supposed to be limited to the US or Europe are found on other continents, e.g., microti and divergens.[91,92]

EU?: A curious Babesia type related to B. odocoilei, a parasite of white-tailed deer, but unrelated to European B. divergens. This human-infecting Babesia has new unreported molecular characteristics.[93]

B. canis: A form of red cell parasite found in dogs which also infects humans.[94]

B. bovis: Another form of Babesia that can infect humans.[95,96]

B. microti: The most common form in the United States, which is often carried by mice.

B. divergens: A form commonly thought of as cattle Babesia, but it also infects humans and is very aggressive. It is the most common Babesia in Europe.

B. equi: A form common in horses but which can infect humans.[97]

B. "unidentified": Increasingly various forms of Babesia are described as "unidentified." This does raise a question about the clinical abilities of some pathologists and the education they are receiving about Babesia. It also raises the issue of how many forms of Babesia species are yet to be identified. Perhaps they are unidentified because they are unique new species.[98-100]

Why Do Multiple Babesia Forms Matter?

A brilliant infectious disease physician who was not feeling well, took a sample of his own blood and found a Babesia-like organism inside a red blood cell. He asked the local lab director to examine this Babesia-like organism. This pathologist said he had "never seen such a thing." Please note that this comment comes from an Ivy League lab director working in New England, where we know that deer ticks have carried Babesia for decades; so this comment was a little scary.

The infected physician took the slide and made images of the infection that was inside of his red blood cells, and mailed them to five of his friends who had experience with Babesia. None were certain what it was, but they all seemed to think it was "some type of Babesia, but not a common one."

The reason I have listed the Babesia forms found in humans above, is so you and your physician will be more educated if your lab realizes they are not looking at mere Babesia microti or Babesia divergens. Further, if you have traveled outside or inside the United States, it might help your physician to know that fact. For example, if your labs come up borderline Lyme-positive and you have been to California and have shortness of breath and strange fevers, it is possible you have Babesia duncani. That species is much more aggressive than Babesia microti, and might require more aggressive treatment.

The simple reality is that some people are infected and do not come up positive using routine testing practices. We might only be diagnosing 1% to 10% of all forms of Babesia in the American population, since all possible Babesia human forms are not part of any lab testing. Indeed if you manage to be tested for Babesia at all, it is a miracle. In my preparation for this book, I only found five physicians who had any idea what I was talking about in terms of cutting-edge 2006 Babesia medicine. All five who were able to converse with me were members of *ILADS,* a group of progressive tick-borne disease specialists who have helped save the lives of my family and many relatives and friends. I contacted some very smart Florida infectious disease physicians, but they assured me that American Babesia was freakishly rare. I have repeatedly diagnosed Babesia in my family members in Florida, the Carolinas and the disastrous Lyme hyper-epidemic states of Pennsylvania and New Jersey.

Indeed, when I was in medical school in Pennsylvania we were told **we should form a diagnosis based on talking carefully to the patient.** In other words, we were supposed to listen first and then get into all the specifics of a patient's troubles. A physical exam and a lab test were meant to add extra data to the working diagnostic options, these were not meant to be the only diagnostic tools. Because I usually treat people who have been seen by as many as 3-25 physicians before me, most patients comment they are surprised we spend one to two hours discussing their illness history. I do this because with many illnesses like Babesia, we are truly in the early stages of understanding, and the symptoms a patient reports help greatly in any diagnosis. We physicians need to be open to learning from, and listening to our patients. Unfortunately, current insurance companies oppose listening by paying 1940's style pay rates, which allow physicians to financially survive only by rushing your care into five-minute sessions. Further, unfortunately some physicians are only able to think as broadly as their blood tests, and function more like lab techs than reflective clinical physicians.

Babesia Life Cycle Simplified

B. micoti is passed to humans usually through a tick bite. It wastes no time in immediately infecting red blood cells. The victim's awareness of the Babesia largely depends on how many red blood cells are infected, how many burst, and perhaps the strain of organism infecting them.

Ticks that carry Babesia in America exist in a wide range of mammals and rodents. The ticks can become infected from feeding on infected deer or other mammals. If a tick feeds on an infected animal, Babesia enters the tick and infects the tick's eggs. These eggs hatch and when the new ticks feed on a different animal, the Babesia reproduces in massive numbers in this newly infected animal.

Malaria Lab Testing Offers Insight In Babesia Testing

Babesia is very similar to malaria and it usually takes a highly trained expert using a microscope to tell them apart. **Both infections enter and infect human red blood cells.**

Let's take a brief look at the status of malaria, an illness that infects 200-500 million people a year and for which the United States has **mandatory reporting requirements,** to see how we are doing before we discuss Babesia lab testing.

To put it bluntly, the use of the microscope worldwide to diagnose this well-established plague is an "imperfect reference standard." The ability to detect malaria requires repeated, ongoing training. The time required to search for malaria in a single smear of blood is often not practical. In England, a **fully-trained microbiologist** missed malaria in 27% of the cases examined.

In another study, glass slides containing thick blood, which is the preferred way to look for malaria, **each took more than two hours to examine.** A special QBC technique was attempted which uses special bright color staining and visualization with ultraviolet light. While it only required about ten minutes per slide, it missed 17% of the positive samples. Perhaps most important in terms of a Babesia application, for which parasites are commonly low in number and can cause no symptoms for a period of time, is that **the QBC test cannot be trusted to find malaria when the quantity of the organism is low.** I believe the same is true of Babesia.[101-104]

In an infectious disease hospital that is accustomed to treating individuals who travel, we see that the type of malaria has a significant role in diagnosis. Japanese physicians **missed 87% of one type of malaria** and missed 22% of another form. Why does this matter? It is stunning to think that a common Asian illness could be missed so commonly in 22-87% of ill patients. And here in America, we have many strains of Babesia and we are not used to treating **any type** of red blood cell infection whatsoever.[105]

In 1994, about 1,000 new cases of malaria were reported to the CDC. Many had a fever or flu-like symptoms after patients returned from a part of the world endemic with malaria. Each person's illness was confirmed by a blood smear and each case was reported to local and/or state health departments. A small number of cases were apparently contracted during blood transfusions and some were acquired locally, e.g., Texas.[106]

Wisely, the Baylor Texas medical center examined 59 patients presenting with malaria in the early 1990's. The lessons learned are worth noting for Babesia, another red blood cell infectious agent that looks similar to malaria under a 1000x microscope. According to the Baylor findings:

- In 25 people, malaria was not considered as an initial diagnosis.

- Five patients came to the hospital with very severe disease. 80% initially received the wrong diagnosis that resulted in increased illness.

- Two patients died despite treatment with malaria medications and blood transfusions.

- One pregnant patient died.

- One baby was infected in utero from its mother.

- Six patients had malaria but had not traveled outside of the United States in over a year.

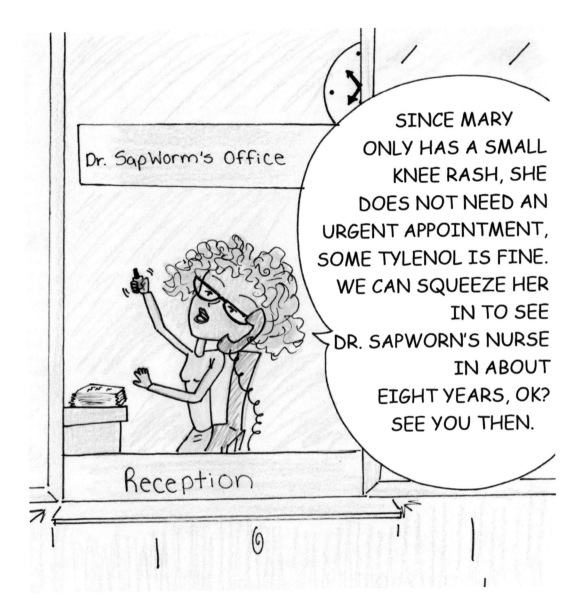

If malaria can be missed as mentioned above, we certainly do not have the knowledge to quickly diagnose Babesia in an overworked, busy common medical office. There they are struggling to pay the massive overhead, office staff and outrageous malpractice insurance.

Baylor's wise conclusions included that malaria in America is either commonly misdiagnosed, or diagnosis is profoundly delayed. Finally, aggressive treatment is not always successful in severe disease.[107]

Babesia Lab Testing and Diagnostic Studies

In medical school if I was taught five minutes about Babesia, I would be surprised. But now tick experts report that in the past 40 to 50 years, as deer and deer ticks explode in numbers and increase their range throughout the United States, this infection has gone from being very rare to being quite common.

Physicians still have a big problem with diagnosis. Most physicians virtually never consider Babesia even when someone clearly has Lyme disease by symptom reporting or positive lab testing. Extensive research and clinical experience shows routine lab testing for both Babesia and Lyme disease are poor. In regards to the two most common Lyme tests, the ELISA and the Western Blot, many labs use inferior test kits that are so poor that they miss patients who present with obvious bulls-eye rashes and clear Lyme symptoms.

If you have a rare bulls-eye rash, you have a spirochete infection like Lyme, period. But large national labs repeatedly fail to detect Lyme in patients with clear bulls-eye rashes, which are considered a certain sign of Lyme (or a very similar infection, Masterson's Disease or STARI). These bulls-eye diagnostic rashes are only seen in 7% of pediatric

Lyme patients (according to Dr. Charles Jones, a Connecticut pediatrician with over 9,000 Tick-illness patients). So diagnosis of tick-borne infections by lab or rash is terrible. I discuss the problems with proper diagnosis in over 200 articles at www.HopeAcademic.com.

My experience as a physician is that sincere and smart allopathic physicians occasionally consider the possibility of Lyme, but virtually **never** diagnose Babesia in routine medical examinations. It is typically only caught by those who have spent **hundreds or thousands of hours specifically studying tick infections.**

After hundreds of hours of study and repeated exposure to Babesia-infected patients, a physician is well equipped at making a clinical diagnosis based solely on talking with the patient and an exam. Occasionally, some types of labs can help make the diagnosis. These include urine tests, antibody tests, visual tests, DNA and other tests.

Urine Tests For Blood

While it is true that some Babesia species cause red blood cell ruptures that are so significant that urine contains significant blood products, this is not a reliable means to diagnose. First, Babesia does not always cause anemia or significant red blood cell rupture. Second, each species has different characteristics and life cycles that are not entirely clear. Third, the test strips used to test for hemoglobin from broken red blood cells are probably not sensitive enough to pick up very low levels of hemoglobin according to the reknowned infectious disease expert of the Carolinas, Dr. Joseph Jemsek and veteran Babesia pathologist Dr. Alan MacDonald.

Nevertheless, on occasion, sixty days of daily testing of your a.m. urine with a hemoglobin dipstick might show a positive. This testing only involves urination at home into a cup. You simply dip the test strip, such as a PerMaxim RediScreen strip into the urine, and read the color next to the container's strip of colors on the side of the container. This test can detect 5-10 red blood cells or their hemoglobin per micro liter.

Antibody Tests

An antibody is a chemical made by your immune system to bind to an invader to remove it. The two classes of antibodies in the core of the body are IgG and IgM. For our purposes, the Ig part stands for an antibody.

So if we were testing for Babesia using an antibody test, you would order a Babesia microti IgG and IgM. But the problem is that many labs are very poor at finding this antibody for many reasons outside the scope of this book. Some labs have spent years perfecting this single test, while others have spent their time on thousands of unrelated tests. Need I say more?

Further, many labs report their findings in terms of "titers," which determines how much infectious antibody is present. Of course, the cutoff point is almost magical. We do not know enough about this illness to have a certain cutoff. Also, these tests usually only search for **one strain** of Babesia—microti.

Visual Tests

In these types of tests, your blood is smeared on a slide and is examined using different stains and special lighting. Some experts in these techniques have told me you can miss the Babesia inside the red blood cells one day, and then see them the following day. Therefore, a blood smear can be highly variable. According to pathologist Dr. Alan MacDonald, many pathologists and lab technicians have not been trained in the special techniques to see Babesia.

DNA Testing

This is the new "hot" lab test and it has some usefulness. But with tick-borne infections it is rather limited. For example, Lyme tissue samples are reliable, but urine and blood samples are almost never positive because Lyme lives within the tissue, and not the blood. Also, some physicians are so enamored with DNA or PCR testing that they will ignore **visible** Lyme in a tissue sample of the gut, brain or muscle, and only trust a DNA sample. DNA tests or PCR testing is only as good as the sample source and only as good as the lab. So detection can be a tricky business.

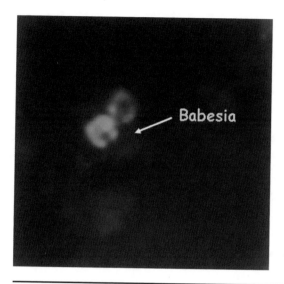

Image (Left): Babesia Positive Blood Smear. A "FISH" test is performed on thin blood smears using an RNA probe to locate active Babesia, which is then visually enhanced with ultraviolet light. Published with permission from Jyotsna Shah, PhD of IGeneX Laboratory in Palo Alto, California.

Fish Testing

This is currently available from IGeneX Labs in Palo Alto, CA, at 800-832-3200 and involves making the most common American Babesia, *(B. microti)*, very visible. Instead of a routine ink-type stain, they use a special probe that sticks to Babesia microti and makes it glow with ultraviolet light.

Immunoblot Antibody Test

Some clinicians seem to feel this might be a potentially useful lab, but some lab experts report it is neither sensitive, nor specific for Babesia. Also, little research exists to demonstrate it has the ability to be standardized.

Three Possible Labs

1) Individuals who have had clear Babesia symptoms found that IGeneX returned the best results to match their clin-

Image (Right):
400x magnification is the only approach many pathologists use in their blood examination. Babesia is hardly easy to see at this magnification.

400x Magnification

1,000x Magnification

1,000x Magnification

Images (Above & Right):
Blood showing Babesia infection, magnified 1,000x with oil.

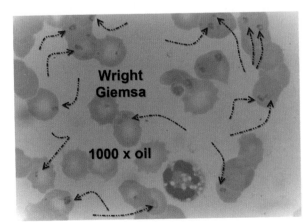

Wright
Giemsa

1000 x oil

Image (Left):
Massive Babesia infection in vast numbers of red blood cells under significant power and after extensive examination.

(Above photos courtesy of Alan MacDonald at St. Catherine of Siena Medical Center in Smithtown, N.Y.)

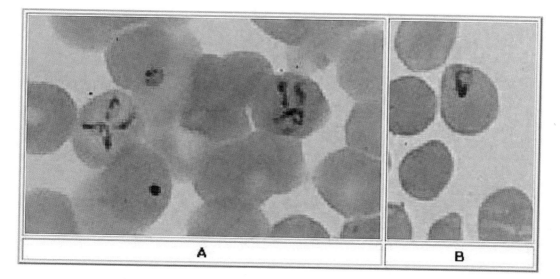

[Babesia microti] [B. divergens] A, B: Infection with *Babesia.* Giemsa stained thin smears. Note in **A**, the tetrad (left side of the image), a dividing form pathognomonic for *Babesia*. Note also the variation in size and shape of the ring stage parasites (compare **A** and **B**), and the absence of pigment. A 6-year-old girl, status post splenectomy for hereditary spherocytosis, infection acquired in the U.S. (Above photo courtesy of the CDC.)

ical picture. This is no surprise because IGeneX's blind New York State testing is exceptional. They are currently testing for Babesia microti and send out the WA-1 Babesia form to another lab of uncertain ability.

2) Dr. J. Whitaker is a famous blood cancer researcher with years of skill in diagnosing abnormal cells. She applies the same knowledge of cell identification in her Bowen Research lab to diagnose Babesia. In these exams, her lab looks for various types of Babesia inside red cells using special techniques. The lab is best at diagnosing B. microti, but is slowly trying to expand their capacity to

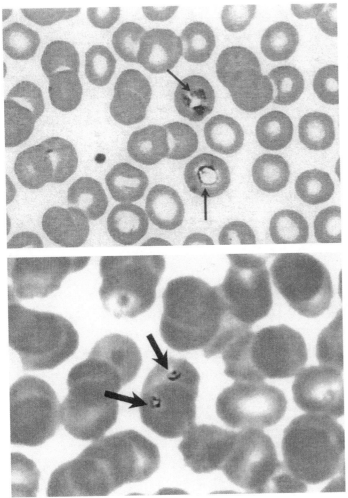

Image (Left):
Trophozoites are the active feeding stage of Babesia. Upper arrow: multiple Trophozoites. Lower arrow: Trophozoite with peripheral nuclear band.

Image (Left):
Compared to the 400x oil image, these highly enlarged images with a careful stain are able to show optimal evaluation of Babesia forms inside of red blood cells. Image shows ring forms in two erythrocytes.

Image (Right):
Traditional stain but very high magnification. Image shows Babesia ring in red blood cell.

(Photos provided courtesy of JoAnne Whitaker, MD, the Bowen Research & Training Institute).

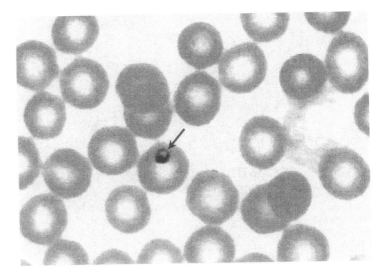

identify other American Babesia forms. However, as any lab performing a visual search, (even one with advanced enhancement techniques), I would consider performing it twice. Dr. Whitaker reports that on some days, Babesia is clearer inside of cells than on other days. In general, my experience is that patients having no symptoms of Babesia are reported as negative by this lab, and patients with a high likelihood of Babesia are commonly diagnosed as positive. I would request a picture of any Babesia infected red blood cells.

3) Medical Diagnostic Labs (MDL) test for Babesia microti using an antibody test and DNA test. Whatever the method, the physician should plan on repeating these tests at least three times before dismissing Babesia, because antibody and DNA testing can miss an infection the first few times. The good news is that many insurance companies have approved of MDL testing.

Other Standard Lab Tests

While most labs are **not** specifically trained to look for Babesia, the following tests might be useful to order:

- A blood smear of peripheral blood with a basic ink Giemsa-stain will occasionally reveal Babesia. However, this test is only as good as the tech performing it and the amount of Babesia present in the drop of blood being examined. If the physician orders only a routine complete blood count (CBC) read by a machine, Babesia inside the red blood cells is more likely to be missed.[108] Be sure to ask the lab to specifically and "manually" perform the following: **"Rule out malaria and hemoprotozoan infection, e.g., Babesia species, Ehrlichia species, Anaplasmas and Bartonella species. Please look at under 1000x with oil. Look for ring forms, tetrads and other signs of parasites."**[109]

Yet even with this request, board-certified Hematologists will miss most parasites within the red blood cells because they will not use oil, won't magnify to 1000x, or be open to the possibility of blood cell parasites. You can only see what you believe possible.

One West Coast research pathologist added to these comments above, and said pathologists or staff members do not see Babesia in a blood smear exam for even more reasons.

- They are trained to look from white cell to white cell. These infection-fighting cells are "where the money is" for them. This is so bad, that in one case of a bone marrow blood sample, 45% of the red blood cells had individual parasites in each of them, and it was missed because pathologists are not trained to look at the red cells—they are in the way, and are skipped over to find the rarer white infection-fighting cells.

- The machine testing is felt to be exceptional and better than they can do manually. And even if they make a slide and an oil exam is asked for at 1000x, it might not be done. A slide with a drop of blood might be made, but when you check it, one feels no oil residue. It seems the machine is trusted more than a human evaluation.

- Stains are chemicals that allow the blood's features to become more visible. Yet the stain chemical can quickly lose its quality in a short time, and some staff do not care, as long as the white cells are clear to see. If the stain is dirty on the slide and red blood cells are not clear, many do not care.

- Some pathologists do not believe in American Babesia, and call the Babesia they might see "platelets" – the part of blood involved in clotting. Babesia and platelets are about the same size.

Nevertheless, despite these common problems, some articles suggest your physician and your pathologist should look for:

a. signs of ruptured red cells (such as urine or blood hemoglobin levels

b. low platelet counts

c. unusual lymphocytes

d. a low white infection cell count (a low WBC level)

e. signs of cells eating red blood cells (hemophagocytosis)

f. pancytopenia or a low number of all the cell types found in blood

g. a urine examination looking for whole red blood cells

and hemoglobin from burst cells

h. ECP stands for eosinophil cationic protein and these might be abnormal in either Babesia or Lyme infections. I am currently researching this test. Quest Diagnostic Labs offers this test with test code 82891N, which is sent to their Nichols Institute Lab.

i.   Babesia can also irritate the liver.

On basic liver tests such as a liver function panel, one can find slightly increased liver cell enzymes leaking out into the blood. Therefore, a lab such as an ALT will be elevated. You might think of the "L" in ALT as representative of the liver. I would also ask for a GGT level, an additional liver test.

Bilirubin is a liver waste product that gives stool its color. It is made from broken down old red blood cells—the same cells that can be infected with Babesia. Bilirubin levels should be tested.

Lactic dehydrogenase or LDH is present in a number of key organs including the liver. Babesia can occasionally alter these levels.

j.   A sedimentation rate (ESR) is a blood test that is sometimes positive with Babesial infection.

k. A Direct Coombs test examines red blood cell clumping and it may or may not be positive.

l.   A finger meter called a "pulse oximeter" can determine if your blood oxygen is too low. Levels are *sometimes* low with very severe Babesia. Levels will be normal in most cases of American Babesia.

m. If a patient has trouble breathing, a chest X-ray or other breathing study may be needed.

The problem with relying on many of the tests above is that only profoundly ill patients will be discovered using these tests. In other words, more than likely these patients will be close to death. Depending upon these tests for the vast majority of Babesia infections will always lead to significant underdiagnosis.

Diagnosis By Co-Infection

If you are trying to locate a few Harley Davidson motorcycle riders, simply follow one around for a few days and you will most likely find others who share a similar love of "Harleys." In the same manner, if you have one tick-borne infection, you will be at a higher risk for finding Babesia and other tick-borne infections. For example, lets say you have lived your entire life in the city of New York. You never go to the suburbs or the great outdoors. Your risk of Babesia is low and your risk of Lyme is low.

However, if you are a hiker, nature walker, gardener, camper, hunter, or if you have a home near woods or wild grasses and shrubs, you are at a high risk for contracting Lyme,

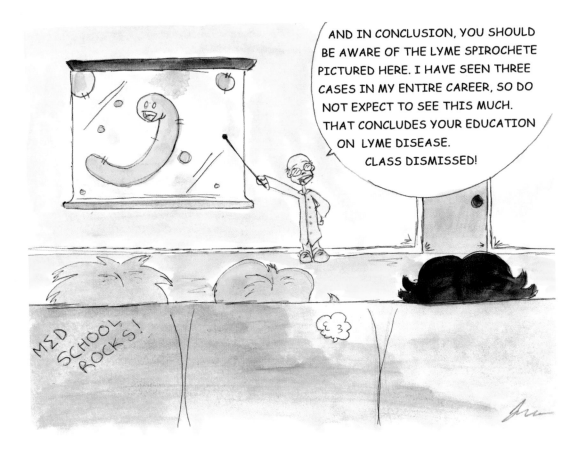

Many smart and talented physicians received virtually no training in diagnosing Lyme or Babesia. And in the rare event they were trained for a few minutes about Babesia microti or Babesia divergens, the odds that they were **trained sufficiently** enough to diagnose it are extremely low.

Bartonella, Anaplasma or Ehrlichia. You are also at a much higher risk of having Babesia. Why is this so?

Any of the infections mentioned above indicates you have been bitten by a tick carrying a disease which affects humans. And since ticks usually carry more than one infection within their stomachs, you are at greater risk for other infections like Babesia.

Therefore, it is important to understand your Babesia testing laboratory options, and consider using labs which have spent time and research to improve their Babesia test methods. Labs such as as IGeneX, MDL and Bowen have focused on tick-borne American infections, and have specifically tried to advance Babesia testing. (Discussing in detail the strengths and weaknesses of each of these labs and other available labs, is outside the scope of this book).

Also if you are positive for one tick infection, Babesia should be considered even if you appear negative on Babesia testing *if you have these symptoms:*

- **High fevers**
- **Dullness**
- **Listless**
- **Chills**
- **Sweats**
- **Headaches**
- **Fatigue**
- **Sleep more than 8 1/2 hours per day**

Lyme and Babesia Combined: What are the symptoms?

When both infections are present, the initial signs and symptoms can be the same, but are often more intense, severe and longer-lasting. Lyme and Babesia attack the body differently, and most clinicians agree that treating both infections is more difficult to treat when simultaneously present.

If You Have Lyme
You are at High Risk For Babesia

I am currently working on a Pediatric Lyme book, so I am not going to get into a great deal of detail about Lyme here. But if you discovered a perfect test for people in America that would accurately diagnose Babesia, almost all people tested will also have Lyme. In the same way, if you discover you have tested positively for Lyme, you should always consider the possibility of Babesia, especially if your Lyme symptoms do not improve with treatment.

What follows below is a type of **diagnosis by association, meaning if you have Lyme or any tick-borne infection, you are at a high risk for Babesia.** Since no lab in the USA can search and find all the forms of Babesia that attack humans, we have to be creative in our search. However, here are three tools you might want to consider using to help diagnose Lyme.

Lyme Checklist

Follows is a simple checklist that was largely derived from a physician having over 14,000 patients with tick-borne infections.[110] If you seem to have some of the symptoms below, you might consider being tested for both Lyme and Babesia.

Do Any of the Following Tick Infection Signs or Symptoms Apply to You?

_____ I lived, visited or vacationed in a high tick-infested area

_____ I participate in outdoor activities such as nature walking, biking, hiking, fishing, gardening, hunting or camping.

_____ I have noticed ticks on my pets or myself.

_____ Other household members or neighbors have Lyme disease.

_____ I remember being bitten by a tick.
When?_____

_____ I remember having the "bull's eye rash."

_____ I have had other skin marks or rashes that did not have a clear cause.

No Lyme check list is complete, because Lyme is the "great imitator" and can cause virtually any medical symptom. But below are some sample common Lyme symptoms.

Circle all numbers you can answer "yes" to, on the next few pages. Some items apply to Lyme and some apply to co-infections.

1) A spotted rash

2) Red streaks

3) Painful fingers with a rash

4) Persistent swollen glands

5) Sore throat

6) Fevers

7) Sore soles, esp. in the a.m.

8) Unexplained back pain

9) Stiffness of the joints or back

10) Muscle pain or cramps

11) Obvious muscle weakness

12) Twitching of the face or other muscles

13) Trouble completing tasks

14) Difficulty thinking

15) Difficulty with concentration

16) Reading is more difficult

17) Problems absorbing new information

18) Word search struggles, name blocking

19) Forgetfulness, poor short-term memory

20) Poor attention

21) Disorientation or getting lost

22) Speech errors such as using a wrong word or misspeaking

23) New typing or writing errors

24) Mood swings, irritability, hostility or depression

25) Unusual eye changes or findings

26) Anxiety or panic attacks

27) Mania or psychosis (hallucinations, delusions, paranoia or a bipolar diagnosis)

28) Tremor

29) Motor or vocal involuntary tics

30) Sensory processing trouble

31) Seizures

32) Headache

33) Light sensitivity

34) Sound sensitivity

35) Joint pain or discomfort in any of the following joints — does not have to be severe or constant:
   a) Fingers, toes
   b) Ankles, wrists
   c) Knees, elbows
   d) Hips, shoulders

36) Vision: double, blurry, unstable prescriptions or floaters

37) Ear pain

38) Hearing: buzzing, ringing or decreased hearing

39) Increased motion sickness, vertigo or spinning feeling

40) Off-balance or "tippy" feeling

41) Lightheadedness, wooziness and unavoidable need

to sit or lie down

42) Tingling, numbness, burning or stabbing sensations or shooting pains

43) Skin hypersensitivity

44) Facial paralysis-Bell's Palsy

45) Dental pain

46) Jaw tenderness and/or pain while chewing

47) Unusual dental decay, abscesses and failed root canals

48) Neck creaks, cracking, stiffness or neck pain

49) Abnormal fatigue, tiredness and decreased stamina

50) Insomnia, fractionated sleep and early awakening

51) Excessive nighttime sleep

52) Napping during the day

53) Unexplained weight gain or loss

54) Unexplained hair loss

55) Pain in genital area

56) Unexplained menstrual irregularity

57) Unexplained milk production or breast pain

58) Irritable bladder or bladder dysfunction

59) Painful, blocked or scarred urinary or genital tissue

60) Erectile dysfunction

61) Loss of libido

62) Queasy stomach or nausea

63) Heartburn, stomach pain

64) Unexplained loose bowel movements or diarrhea

65) Constipation

66) Low abdominal pain, cramps

67) Heart murmur, valve prolapse or valve damage

68) Heart palpitations, skipped or missed beats

69) "Heart block" on EKG

70) Chest wall pain or rib soreness

71) Foggy thinking

72) Breathlessness or "air hunger"

73) Unexplained chronic cough

74) Night sweats

75) Exaggerated symptoms or worse hangover from alcohol

76) Symptom flares every 4 weeks

77) Symptom flares with antibiotic use

78) Decreased speech speed and smoothness

79) Decreased coordination, e.g., walking heel-to-toe with your eyes closed

Lyme enters the brain within hours to days and causes many personality and mood changes. In the manner that the brain is vulnerable to the absence of oxygen or blood sugar after only a few minutes, the brain is very sensitive to Lyme.

Here are additional symptoms adding to those mentioned briefly above. *Any* **psychiatric problem and any personali-**

ty problem can be enhanced or caused by Lyme. This is a fact that is not appreciated in most psychology and psychiatry circles, due to a lack of education and awareness about Lyme.

Unfortunately this lack of awareness to Lyme's effects on personality can cause serious relational trouble and under-treated mental illness. Psychiatric problems require creative approaches when their cause is Lyme and depression, or Lyme and anxiety. Dosing and medications often require a unique approach when Lyme is the cause of the emotional struggle.

Everyday Observations of Tick-Borne Illness

- Poor self-awareness and poor insight
- Moody and irritable
- Rigidity
- Impulsivity
- Catastrophic reactions to mild or modest irritations
- Eccentric obsessiveness
- New distractibility which was not present as a five-year old
- New trouble finishing tasks which was not present when healthy
- Acting unwisely with money, drinking, drugs, sex or speech content
- Stress with transitions or change
- Primitive emotions
- Excessive entitlement

- Expecting overly special treatment from people around you
- Routine lateness
- Empathic deficits
- Deficits in perception of personal social skills
- Poor boundary awareness
- "Flaky" or "spacey"
- "Clueless" about self health
- Blow ups and excess anger
- Reduced frustration tolerance
- Rigidity to new ideas, changes, demands on time
- Narcissism and/or profound self-centered thinking
- Poor ability to process trauma
- Eccentric personality traits
- Wired intensity
- Organizational extremes – sloppy or must have profound order
- Regressed feelings and thoughts – excess sensitivity to being heard, cared for and respected
- Dead creativity
- Rage or mania

Reading the Western Blot Correctly

Currently, it seems that the majority of expert Lyme physicians who are treating and researching tick-borne illnesses are unhappy with the ELISA test. Dr. Charles Ray Jones, who has treated 10,000 children with many types of tick infection, believes the ELISA is a terrible screening test because it misses large numbers of patients. Other physicians also regard it as nearly useless.

Instead, the Western Blot test is the preferred choice of many Lyme experts such as Dr. Jones. But just like an automobile, the quality of the Western Blot can range from poor to excellent. A good quality Western Blot uses more than one Lyme strain, and also collects diverse proteins from these strains in equal amounts. This type of Western Blot test is rarely performed.

According to Dr. Jones, what is important is to look for "fingerprint bands" within the Western Blot result. A fingerprint band simply means that you have a positive band or antibodies against a **highly specific and unique protein of Lyme** that is not found in other organisms.

The Western Blot lists the antibodies that are produced by the body in response to the Lyme bacteria. The map separates these antibodies by weight and reports them as units called *kilo daltons*, or kDa. There are nine proteins specific for Lyme and they are:

18
23
23-25 (Some labs combine these two proteins)
31
34
37
39
83
93
83-93 (Some labs combine these two proteins)

According to Dr. Charles Jones, if you have even **one** of these bands present, you have been exposed to Lyme, period. You will notice that many labs have very few test proteins not included in the full list above. Simply put, most labs offer incomplete and unacceptable Lyme testing. And since we now know that Lyme changes its outer surface proteins very rapidly once it enters the human body, (and does so repeatedly), more thorough testing becomes necessary.

Many labs try to remove the physician's ability to think and merely report a "positive" or "negative" band. Yet I want to know about any shades of gray or borderline readings. If you have a "borderline" or "indeterminate" result for one of these bands, it does not mean your result is negative, it just means that the band's size was not big and dark enough to call it a clear and certain positive. But the test is seeing something in the positive region. For example, lets say your 31 band was "IND" or indeterminate. It means the tech saw a mild line of antibodies binding to a specific protein from the Lyme bacteria. IND also means that the line was not as dark as the "positive control."

What is a positive control? It is a check on the accuracy of the test. Smart labs know mistakes can happen so they run a "control" to make sure the test was done correctly. So a positive control sample has all the Lyme proteins being tested and all should show up positive. A negative control has no Lyme specific proteins and should never show a reaction or band. Personally, I believe the IND's or indeterminates are weak positives.

Lyme DNA or PCR Testing

The problem with DNA testing of Lyme is that the best results are received from **tissue** samples, such as bone marrow samples, intestinal biopsies, skin biopsies or muscle biopsies. Lyme generally does not live within urine or blood. So the odds of finding DNA samples of Lyme in bodily fluids are low. Some labs such as MDL are covered by insurance and will allow the clinician to *repeatedly* look for this DNA within blood samples.

Many blood tests can become abnormal when in the presence of Lyme or Babesia. You can discuss with your physician which labs to consider. Lyme and Babesia alter the results of many inflammation and even rare hormone tests that are almost never considered, e.g., specialized thyroid antibodies, Free Testosterone, Testosterone, DHEA, MSH, and T3 Thyroid levels. These tests can be more sensitive than some Lyme or Babesia labs, which again, are often only positive in severe illness.

Babesia Lab Testing: A Conclusion

Many tick experts report that in the past 40 to 50 years Babesia infection has grown from being very rare to being much more common. Despite the time lapse, we still have a problem with diagnosis. First, most physicians do not consider Babesia unless someone first tests positive for Lyme disease. Research documents show that the two most common Lyme tests, the

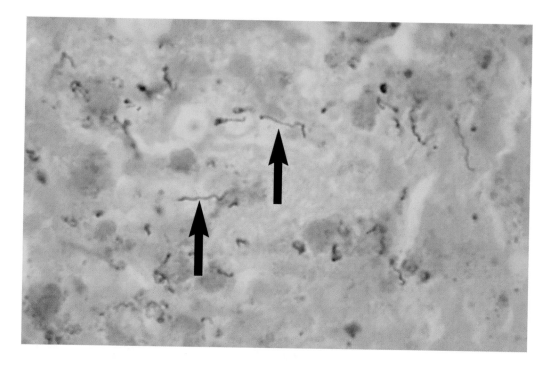

Blood, urine and spinal fluid tests for Lyme disease are notoriously unreliable, according to blind samples sent to many laboratories. Biopsies often offer much more useful and clearer results, if a pathologist is willing to take the time to search for an extended time. This patient was unable to be successfully treated. But then, only after this biopsy with obvious Lyme spirochetes, was the patient able to begin the healing of his raw intestinal tract.   (Image courtesy of Dr. Martin Fried, Jersey Shore University Medical Center)

ELISA and the Western Blot, when performed at routine labs, are often unreliable. Some labs clearly use inferior Lyme test kits. These kits are as cheap as the cheap payments given to the lab to perform them, and fail to diagnose patients with obvious bulls-eye rashes and clear Lyme symptoms. I discuss this problem and other Lyme issues in over 200 articles available at www.personalconsult.com.

In summary, my experience is that a Babesia diagnosis is as rare as a unicorn mainly because the lab testing and diagnostic awareness for Babesia is absolutely terrible. While Lyme is diagnosed more often than is Babesia, the cases which manage to be reported are only a small fraction of people with real infections.

Finally, I believe that sincere and smart physicians almost never diagnose Babesia because it is highly specialized medicine. ***Babesia is typically only diagnosed by those who have spent hundreds or thousands of hours studying tick-borne infections.*** It is a type of highly specialized medicine similar to treating HIV or AIDS patients. Meaning, most physicians have not taken the time to master the massive complexity of AIDS treatment, and those that do, end up with large numbers of AIDS patients.

Babesia Treatment

Babesia and malaria are not identical parasites, but they do have much in common. One reason for the slow progress in Babesia research and treatment is due to the distinction between veterinary and medical parasitology. Babesia is perceived as more of an **animal** infection while malaria is a profound **human** infection. This division, when it comes to Babesia, is entirely false. Both organisms infect human red blood cells and are treated with the same types of medications.[111]

In this chapter I will introduce you to real clinical experts in Babesia treatment. We will learn their treatment options and discuss cutting-edge information about an anti-Babesia herb. Then I will list all the major Babesia medications currently available and briefly summarize new research, practical issues, effectiveness, dosing and side effects.

Babesia Medications

Malaria is one of the most serious worldwide health problems, with at least 300 million people becoming infected each year. Babesia is similar to malaria in that both enter red blood cells. Most medications for Babesia were first used for malaria, so if you read educational handouts on the medications that follow, you might be surprised to notice Babesia is never mentioned. Despite this, the effectiveness of malarial medicines for the treatment of Babesia is utilized by many experts having different treatment styles and philosophies.

While the patient should rely upon the advice of their treating physician, some experts on killing tick-borne infections have been kind enough to offer me some of their thoughts. As you will see, the treatment of Babesia co-infections is still evolving and becoming more effective each year. The material below does not do justice to the broad approaches many experts use, but is only offered as an introduction. All the treatments offered by the four experts listed below are discussed in detail later in this book along with new research, side effects, interactions and other critical information.

Routine Traditional Babesia Treatments

Option 1:   Mepron 750 mg two times per day with
                   Zithromax 250-600 mg per day for
                   7-10 days

Option 2:   Clindamycin 600 mg every 6 hours with
                   Quinine 650 mg every 8 hours for 7-10 days

Child Option: Clindamycin 5 mg/kg every 6 hours and
                   Quinine 8.3 mg/kg every 8 hours for
                   children.[112]

Approximately one-third of the patients taking these combinations stop treatment due to uncomfortable side effects. The primary concern of some Babesia experts with this traditional treatment approach is that chronic Babesia is not completely killed within 10 days. The goal of those who embrace this traditional approach is not to use medications too long that may have side effects and carry possible risks.

Joseph Burrascano, MD (New York State)

Dr. Burrascano treated Lyme and Babesia from 1983 until 2006 when he retired from clinical medicine to pursue other medical goals such as tick infection research. He was personally infected at the age of 13, and since no physician was able to diagnose him, he remained infected until the 1980's when progressive Lyme research began and he himself began treatment and treating others. Since tick-borne infections are virtually ignored in medical school and residencies, he had to invent many treatment protocols for both Lyme and Babesia infections.

You might think the State Medical Board would value his expertise after treating more than 14,000 patients from all over the world. Instead, his thanks for saving thousands of lives and giving away all of his protocols for free, was that the State Medical Board of New York and some non-clinical Ivy League types continually tried to destroy his career. As they abused him for his successful treatment approaches, the New York Medical Board ignored over 60 citizen complaints against physicians who offered very conservative treatment.

While Babesia was never part of the New York Medical Board's abuse allegations, after years of educating them about other tick-borne infections like Lyme, they concluded their costly harassment with **no written criticisms of either his diagnoses or treatments.** The board determined that this medical and science debate had no place within the disciplinary jurisdiction of the medical board.

To many, Dr. Burrascano is considered the Father of modern clinical Lyme treatment. While Ivy League physicians were telling patients they were "just fine," or "crazy" for thinking they were not cured after 21 days of antibiotics, Dr. Joe was treating them as long as was required to effect a cure for their Lyme.

In addition to Lyme, "Dr. Joe" has also been concerned about Babesia infections for decades. Why does this matter to him? Simply, if one reads the available studies on human Babesia infections in the United States, it is clear that most of these articles are approximately ten years old or newer. This means that the material on United States Babesia is very new, and the number of articles is very limited. Perhaps because of the poverty of articles and lack of experience in diagnosing Babesia, many sincere infectious disease physicians are only very recently aware of Babesia. In contrast, Dr. Joe has been treating Babesia since 1983.

Dr. Joe Burrascano is aware of traditional Babesia treatments, but feels that these short-term malaria treatments often do not apply to curing established chronic Babesia. For example, while early and acute Babesia can sometimes be successfully treated with three weeks of Mepron and Zithromax, he has found that entrenched chronic Babesia requires at least five months of continual treatment. This treatment duration approximates the four-month life cycle of the red blood cell— the cells in which Babesia thrive.

He explains that Babesia is a Piroplasm and not a bacteria. It is a tiny parasite that requires special treatment. This means that medications focused on killing Lyme bacteria will usually fail to remove Babesia because it is not a bacteria. It is a parasite that lives in red blood cells.

Dr. Burracano feels that if a Lyme patient has been extensively treated and yet remains ill, the doctor and patient should seriously suspect a Babesia co-infection.

Just as in Lyme disease, the longer one has been infected with Babesia, the longer the treatment that will be required. The treatment duration should not be some cliché cookbook amount of time, but should include clinical improvement to the point of a cure.

Dr. Burrascano's Treatment Options: Babesia Plan A

Dr. Joe believes the most effective treatment for Babesia to be Mepron (atovaquone) at 750 mg per teaspoon twice a day taken with a fatty meal, along with Zithromax (azithromycin) at 600 mg daily. The Zithromax is to prevent resistance to Mepron. "Resistence" is the ability of the infection to develop genes that make a medication useless. Mepron taken alone has a 20% failure rate due to the development of resistance. When one adds Zithromax, the resistance rate falls to nearly zero.

Since most physicians believe more Babesia is killed during simultaneous treatments, he also adds some form of Sweet

Wormwood or Sweet Annie (Artemisia or Artemisinin) to the treatment regimen. If a patient has access to a very high-quality form of Artemisia (such as at a health food store), the dose is 500 mg three times a day. Alternately one can use a high-quality standardized form of Artemisinin at 100 three times a day.

Dr. Joe has noticed some patients on a Mepron/Zithromax regimen have a "die-off reaction" or a Herxheimer-like reaction that occurs on day four and also during the fourth week of therapy. It is unknown if this process is due to a die-off of Babesia or Lyme disease.

Another reason Dr. Joe treats for five months is because many patients have continual and significant fevers, chills or sweats until around five months of treatment. This information would seem to support the red blood cell four-month life span hypothesis. Another reason for routinely treating Babesia for five months is based on his relapse research. Simply, if some infected red blood cells are left behind, then the infection can reoccur or persist, causing a relapse. When he compared his success rate and relapse rate, it seemed to clearly indicate that **five months was more successful than four months**. Perhaps this is because Mepron has such a long half-life, taking three weeks to achieve therapeutic levels. Most of the first month of treatment is devoted to raising blood levels.

The most common problems typically experienced with Mepron are diarrhea, mild nausea and the expense of Mepron,

(Mepron costs $856.00 **wholesale** for 210 mls, or 20 days of treatment). Therefore, if cost is a concern, he may instead prescribe Lariam at 250 mg, once every five days for five months. Some physicians believe you should "load" Lariam within the first week with a higher dose, but Dr. Joe feels the side effects are too harsh for some patients.

Another Babesia treatment option is Malarone. Malarone contains 250 mgs of the active agent of Mepron, (atovaquone), in addition to proquanil. He prescribes three Malarone 250 mg tablets twice daily, which is equivalent to 750 mg of Mepron twice a day. However, since Mepron in pill form is generally only about 50% absorbed, and if it is not taken with a fatty meal, the blood levels also fall markedly. Malarone also contains proquanil which might reduce resistence and increase effectiveness.

Dr. Joe has had few problems with other medications interacting during these treatments. However, he did mention that simultaneously taking a common Lyme antibiotic, doxycycline, lowers Mepron levels significantly.

Mepron binds very tightly to blood cells carrying proteins. So this feature can radically change blood levels of some common medications. For example, the antibiotic Rifampin levels with Mepron causes Mepron levels to fall and Rifampin levels to rise significantly.[113]

The Lyme biotoxin binder, Questran (cholestyramine), is also not prescribed by Dr. Joe at the same time as Mepron, since the cholestyramine might bind the Mepron within the bile and lower the body's blood level. (It is unknown whether Welchol, chitosan, charcoal, or detox clays would also lower Mepron, but it is a possibility).

Further, Dr. Joe thinks it is wise to test the blood level for Mepron. This can be performed by LabCorp and forwarded to Focus Technologies, the lab that actually checks the blood levels. I think this process is very wise, since I have found patients to have a very wide range of drug levels in their blood. While some patients can have blood levels that are therapeutically useless, others have levels that are far too high. It is important to obtain an objective level instead of guessing.

Both the Lariam and Malarone are dosed for five months. The only concern about the former, Lariam, is that it does not penetrate as deeply into the tissues as Mepron does. Therefore, Lariam only controls and limits Babesia that is located in the blood. Therefore, Lariam is better as a control agent than as a curative one.

Mepron can rarely cause a temporary yellowish discoloration of the vision. Regular blood counts (CBC's) and liver panels (LFT's) are recommended during any prolonged course of therapy with any of these agents. Patients who are not cured after this treatment plan can be retreated, but with higher doses of Mepron. This has proven effective for many of Dr.

Burrascano's patients, especially large individuals or those whose treatment fails with lower doses. Testing medication blood levels can show the need for higher dosing in a retrial.

Dr. Burrascano's Plan B

If the Mepron protocol appears to fail in a patient, then Dr. Joe switches to **Malarone** at three pills twice daily, and adds Bactrim, Flagyl or Zithromax.

- Bactrim DS (or Septra DS) is taken at one dose, twice a day

- Flagyl ER (extended release) is dosed at 750 mg ER tablets twice a day.

Zithromax, Biaxin or Ketek is also added. Dr. Joe appreciates that there is no available research on these other agents other than Zithromax use in combination with Mepron, but he has found some success adding them to the medications listed above.

Dr. Burrascano's Plan C

Another option is the use of **Lariam** 250 mg tablets, taken every five days in combination with Zithromax, Biaxin, or Ketek, with the possible addition of doxycycline and Flagyl.

All supposedly can increase Lariam's effectiveness.

Treating Babesia forms that are not B. microti

Most diagnosed forms of American Babesia are actually Babesia microti. Dr. Joe's experience is unique in that he is very aware that some of his patients have forms of Babesia that are not Babesia microti. For example, he has had to treat Babesia divergens and WA1. He reports these are tough infections that require aggressive treatment.

Dr. Joe is dialoguing with some physicians who do not use Mepron, but rather use the antimalaria herb Artemisinin combined with Flagyl, Bactrim, Doxycycline and Zithromax. Dr. Joe's initial impression is that patient results are generally not very good without the use of Mepron.

Dr. Burrascano's Treatment-Resistance Options

While Dr. Burrascano has studied the traditional protocol that prescribes Clindamycin, 600 mg four times a day, with Quinine, 650 mg four times a day, he is not pleased with this option. Why? His experience is that the suggested two weeks of treatment is nearly impossible to tolerate due to hearing loss, rash, fever and headaches. Treatment failures can also occur.

Dr. Burrascano believes those who clearly fail other treatments should consider Gentamicin. He believes this can be a powerful medication in humans for treating a wide range of infections including Babesia. It is currently already successfully used to treat livestock infected with piroplasms. But he has only heard anecdotal reports of Gentamicin benefit in people. For example, some preliminary studies report two weeks of treatment at standard Gentamicin doses has proven effective during early disease. However, he cautions that we do not have much information about the effectiveness of Gentamicin on late and advanced cases of Babesia, and the optimal dose and duration is unclear. Further, the main side effect of concern with Gentamicin is a risk of hearing loss, and the discomfort and risk of an injection or an IV tube.

Years ago, daily Pentamidine shots were used, but Dr. Burrascano does not suggest using this treatment because it causes severe pain in addition to abscesses and permanent scars on the buttocks. Patients may also suffer from a risk of glucose intolerance. Further, he is displeased with its effectiveness, so he feels it a poor choice for the treatment of Babesia.

Dr. Joseph Jemsek, (N. Carolina)

This infectious disease expert is one of the top tick-borne infection clinicians in the United States. He is easily the most well-informed and experienced Lyme and Babesia expert in the Carolinas. He was the first physician to diagnose

HIV/AIDS in this part of the country, proving him a leader in diagnosing new infections. Dr. Jemsek never treats two patients in the exact manner, but he was willing to offer some basic information.

Dr. Jemsek feels that Babesia treatment is fairly new and physicians need to be flexible in modifying their treatments as more data and clinical experience appears. The proper treatment options in 2006 will possibly be different in 2007.

His first lesson for clinicians is the importance of accepting that in the United States, Babesia routinely exists with Lyme infection. He also theorizes that it might be possible for some patients to only have Babesia, such as a mild form of Babesia microti, and not display any symptoms. If such people existed but who were otherwise healthy and had a good spleen, they might be functional without any treatment. However, in the United States, symptomatic Babesiosis is virtually always combined with symptomatic Lyme disease. When Babesia and Lyme are both present in your body, it presents a real problem.

Why is this so? Lyme weakens your immune system and makes it less capable of controlling Babesia. Interestingly, Babesia infection helps make Lyme disease stronger. Dr. Jemsek feels that these two infections working together as a team are tough on the body. One infection plus another infection leads to sicker patients.

His second thought is that Babesia is generally best diagnosed through **clinical experience.** While some labs are able to diagnose it, many forms are not even tested for and many labs struggle to diagnose them. Dr. Jemsek tracks common symptoms that are attributable to Babesia. He searches for these prominent but routine Babesia symptoms in his patients:

- **Significant fatigue**

- **Night sweats or sweating during the day**

- **Fever**

- **Chills**

While these signs may overlap with Bartonella or other co-infections, these symptoms seem to be **more pronounced in a person infected with Babesia.**

While these signs can also exist to some degree with Lyme infection, in Dr. Jemsek's experience, if they are caused by Lyme alone, they seldom last beyond days or weeks. Conversely with Babesia, these complaints are more prominent and are present after a month of illness.

Dr. Jemsek treats Babesia in three ways, depending upon the patient's symptoms. If one seems to be mild or moderately ill, he will use the following treatment option.

Dr. Jemsek's Mild-Moderate Babesia Treatments

- Mepron 750 mg (teaspoon) twice a day with a fatty meal

- Zithromax 500 mg twice a day

- He has patients take this for 5-7 days per week for 6-8 weeks.

At times he may replace Zithromax with Ketek. The Ketek is dosed at 400 mg tablets, (two at bedtime), so any possible blurred vision happens while you are sleeping. He never combines Zithromax and Ketek together in any treatment plan because they interact.

Most patients can take a holiday week after treatment week three or four from Mepron and Zithromax combined.

Patients are also treated with a Lyme cyst or "seed" killer from the *imidazole* medication class. Specifically, either Flagyl (metronidazole) or Tindamax (tinidazole) 500mgs twice a day is prescribed during the last 3-5 consecutive days before their holiday week.

Why use cyst-killers when one is treating Babesia? Lyme should not be ignored just because one is treating Babesia, particularly when treatments are available for both Lyme and Babesia that will slow Lyme's activity and are *"bacteriostatic"* (Zithromax, Ketek and Biaxin). These medications will typically not kill the active forms during this treatment period. Lyme has many different forms at all times. Some are active and some are less active (cystic). If one started treatment by killing Lyme before Babesia, which is what most tick-infection experts do, than the Lyme that is still remaining in your body may be:

1) resistant to common antibiotics

2) a tough minority Lyme strain or

3) a theoretically protected cyst form

Two medications, Flagyl and Tindamax, are believed to kill the cystic forms. So while the Zithromax might increase protective cyst forms, Flagyl and Tindamax will kill them. Dr. Jemsek calls this a "stun and kill" approach. One uses antibiotics that kill active forms and which promote stunned spirochetes into becoming cysts, and then cyst killers like Flagyl and Tindamax are used.

In some patients, Dr. Jemsek also uses the antimalaria herb Artemisinin beginning with 300 mg twice a day, and then rapidly increasing to 900 mg twice a day within a week or less. This regimen may be added during different aspects of Babesia treatment. The total dosage result is 30 mg/kilogram per day. This daily dose is divided into two doses. To calculate your daily dose, use one of these conversion tools:

A kilogram x 2.2 = your weight in pounds:

$$\frac{pounds}{2.2} = kilograms$$

So a 150-pound person would be calculated this way:

$$\frac{150 \text{ pounds}}{2.2} = \text{kilograms}$$

68.2 kilograms = kilogram answer

68 kilograms x 30 kilograms per day equals 2,040 mg of artemisinin each day or approximately 1000 mg twice a day.

Dr. Jemsek's Moderate to Severely Ill Treatments

Either because Lyme, Bartonella and Babesiosis infections may limit intestinal absorption of medications or because Babesia medications may cause excessive intestinal side effects, this Jemsek approach uses IV treatments. First, the doctor and the patient both need to agree that an IV approach is preferred for various reasons, e.g., the Babesia is causing serious neurological and cognitive problems. The IV approach is:

- IV Clindamycin 900 mg every 12 hours for 8 weeks (5-7 days per week). Patients are given IV holidays based on many factors, and here are some patterns Dr. Jemsek uses, including one or two weeks off:

  a. IV medication for 3 weeks, off a week, then on 3 final weeks

b. IV medication for 4 weeks, off a week, then on 4 final weeks

c. IV medication for 2 weeks, off a week, then on 2 weeks, then off a week, and then 2 final weeks. This last approach is reserved for patients who experience significant side effects or bacterial die-off.

Important Add-ons to IV Clindamycin

- Mepron 750 mg (one teaspoon twice daily taken with a fatty meal) or Malarone 250 mg dosed at 2-3 tablets twice a day.

- IV Zithromax 500 mg once daily

- Artimisinin is begun at 300 mg twice a day, and then rapidly increased to 700-900 mg twice a day during a week. This dosing is commonly used for seven weeks (with a one-week break) and rarely fourteen weeks (with a one-week break every 4 weeks).

In order to keep the Lyme in check while treating Babesia, Dr. Jemsek adds either Flagyl or Tinidazole, 500 mg tablets twice daily for 3-5 days during the last treatment week (e.g., week 3 or 4) in the treatment cycle, if tolerated. The reasons for this were discussed above. Generally since this program is effective at killing Lyme cysts, patients will feel ill during the Lyme cyst die-off so this regimen is not followed for more than five days, and can be as few as two days if this is all the patient can tolerate.

Once a patient ends this aggressive IV Babesia treatment, Dr. Jemsek does not ignore Babesia. While he is choosing medications to kill Lyme or other tick-borne infections, he does include agents likely to have some mild to modest Babesia activity such as the related antibiotics, Ketek and Zithromax. (We know that Zithromax has some ability to kill malaria, and virtually all approaches against Babesia began as malaria medications).

Dr. Jemsek's Approach to Chronic and Resistant Babesia

If a patient is still showing residual signs of Babesia, such as significant sweating, he attempts this treatment:

Lariam 250 mg with 4-5 tablets loaded during the first week, followed by one tablet per week following this loading dose.

- Doxycycline 200 mg twice a day

- Bactrim DS or Septra DS (sulfa medications) in the double-strength forms to equal 800 mg of sulfamethoxazole and 160 mg of trimethoprim. For example, a man or women weighing 150-160 pounds would take 1-1/2 to 2 DS (double strength) tablets twice a day.

- Zithromax 500 mg twice a day or Ketek 400 mg, two at bed time, or Mepron at 750 mg (teaspoon) twice per day taken with a fatty meal.

Since he is still concerned with Lyme while treating Babesia, he pulses Flagyl or Tindamax 5-7 days per week, but sometimes settles for 3 or 4 days a week, since both of these medications are difficult for the patient to take due to side effects or Lyme die-off reactions.

Dr. Richard Horowitz, (New York State)

Dr. Horowitz is a well-rounded and brilliant clinician who has an excellent national reputation for creative and custom-tailored medical care. He has been both treating and researching Babesia treatments for many years. Below we illustrate some important highlights of his Babesia treatments. He was most concerned to make it understood that Lyme is rarely the only infection passed on during a tick bite. He points out that many studies show ticks carry vast numbers of infections within their stomach and saliva. Therefore, he feels **physicians and patients need to understand co-infections are the norm and not the exception.** So while he is offering some Babesia treatment options, he feels it important to point out that Lyme, Bartonella and other tick-borne infections must simultaneously be addressed for optimal treatment.

Further, in clinical treatment a patient is seen approximately every four weeks, and based on their complaints, the treatment is altered in order to address the infection causing the greatest trouble, which might not be Babesia. So what follows are treatment suggestions, and not pages from a simple cookbook, since no patient is ever treated in exactly the same manner.

Dr. Horowitz explained that while Babesia can have many symptoms, many of these symptoms overlap with other infections. For example, Babesia can cause headaches, joint pain and muscle aches, but so can other tick-borne infections. He tends to note symptoms such as **chills, fevers and sweats** to track Babesia, understanding that these can be present during other tick infections, but tend to be prominent in active Babesia. Also, since some of these symptoms can be caused by other medical problems such as perimenopause, we should not be simplistic in thinking that the sole cause of fevers, chills and sweats is Babesia. A good work up for any medical problem includes using traditional and integrative medicine to examine other causes of your symptoms. Further, many serious medical conditions cause fevers, chills and sweats, such as Tuberculosis and Non-Hodgkin's Lymphoma, so these need to be ruled out before rigidly limiting treatment to tick-borne infections.

The Horowitz Core Initial Babesia Treatments for Adults

• Mepron 750 mg liquid taken as two teaspoons, twice a day and with a fatty meal (for patients over 120 pounds).

- Zithromax 250 mg twice a day (to decrease resistance to Mepron).

- Septra or Bactrim Double Strength (DS) tablets one, twice a day. This is a "Sulfa" medication that can have side effects. Dr. Horowitz has studied a wide range of doses up to four DS per day. Four per day caused a high number of side effects that was unacceptable for treatment.

- Dr. Horowitz uses the antimalaria herb artemisinin. Please see my book on artemisinin and Artemisia on Amazon.com or on www.HopeAcademic.com. Dr. Horowitz uses artemisinin 100 mg dosed as one to three capsules three times a day (300 mg-900 mg per day). He has used forms that are carefully controlled for purity such as Allergy Research Group's brand, and has recently been using Dr. Zhang's formulation of Artemisiae. His reasoning is simply that Dr. Zhang has exceptional expertise in malaria and Babesia-related herbs such as artemisinin. Further, Chinese medicine has extensively treated malaria because it has been a long and serious medical problem in Asia. As said before, most antimalaria medications also seem to have anti-Babesia properties. Dr. Zhang's web site is www.sinomedresearch.org. He uses Hepapro company to make his herbs. Hepapro is the exclusive maker of Dr. Zhang's herbs and they can be contacted by phone at 888-788-4372 or Hepapro@hotmail.com.

Dr. Horowitz and I defer you to Dr. Zhang's highly respected products and writings because Dr. Zhang adds some other important herbs to his Artemisiae product to treat Babesia. Dr. Zhang generally uses these herbal treatments for 30-90 days depending on the patient's response to treatment. In another section of this book I go into great detail about various forms of Artemisia such as artemisinin. I explain that the large fern Artemisia can yield weak artemisinin or more potent synthetic **artesunate**. Synthetic artesunate is felt to be able to kill more malaria and Babesia due to its increased potency, but it still leaves the body fast enough to limit side effects. Dr. Zhang's Artemisiae is actually strong and potent artesunate. In a later section, I offer extended information on the various forms of medicines derived from Artemisia.

While some articles seem to imply the possibility of hearing trouble or brainstem effects from taking artemisinin or related products, Dr. Horowitz has never seen any of these problems with artemisinin. And quite to the contrary, if a patient is dizzy or has some brain fog, the treatment seems to help with these problems.

Dr. Horowitz's Stage Two Treatment

As a trend, the treatment listed above is often clinically effective.

But if it proves ineffective because a strain of Babesia is not vulnerable, or if the patient has improved to the point where they have no significant sweats, chills or high fever for approximately 4-8 weeks, then Dr. Horowitz will adjust his treatment to kill other infections, but will also continue to address residual Babesia.

One option is to replace his initial Mepron approach with Malarone, which contains low dose Mepron (atovaquone) with proquanil. A commonly prescribed tablet size is 250 mg of Mepron with 100 mg of proquanil. Generally, to keep any residual Babesia in check, he will prescribe a Malarone 250 mg tablet per day. This low dose can be used along with virtually all medications. If he is trying to attack Lyme, Ehrlichia, or Bartonella, the Malarone will not undermine these treatments. He will use the Malarone as long as the patient continues to have symptoms such as fever, chills and sweats outside the modest range of other tick-borne infections. His duration of treatment could be six weeks to six months depending on whether the patient has virtually no Babesia symptoms or ongoing residual and troublesome fever, severe fatigue, chills and sweats.

Generally one looks for some improvement and ultimately the resolution of symptoms. Further, repeating three Babesia baseline lab tests from IGeneX can sometimes be helpful in tracking improvement. The IFA, PCR and FISH tests are useful for this purpose. Specifically, the IFA is an antibody test designed to detect Babesia antibodies. If antibodies are present they will appear as fluorescent. The PCR machines are able to take the smallest, invisible fragments of Babesia and grow Babesia DNA to a quantity that can be detected. The FISH test uses a special sticky Babesia-specific fluorescent material that makes the infection glow under UV magnification. While some patients with active Babesia can test negatively in a high number of cases, these tests can be somewhat useful in tracking overall improvement.

Dr. Horowitz's Stage Three Treatment

If these two treatment options fail, Dr. Horowitz considers the possibility of a **resistant form** of Babesia or else the treatment is simply not a good fit to kill this specific form of Babesia. At this point he will use the following options:

- Lariam 250 mg every 5-7 days

- Plaquinel 200 mg twice a day

- Doxycycline 200 mg twice per day

Lariam 250 mg is taken every 5-7 days. He has found that his 700-800 patients treated with Lariam have **not had** the dramatically publicized side effects such as severe psychiatric problems—suicide, psychosis, etc. He thinks this may be because he does not "load" the Lariam, using five pills within the first week as a "loading" dose. This technique is initiated when treating active malaria. He feels that in Babesia treatment, this loading can cause too many side effects. He tells patients to halt their Lariam and contact him if they feel uncomfortable with the side effects.

Dr. Horowitz does not believe that Lariam fully kills Babesia, but that it will simply hold it in check, which is often enough for continued good health. In terms of Plaquenil and Doxycycline, Dr. Horowitz feels these have merit because of past successes in India when common malaria medications were unavailable and these were used instead.

Dr. Horowitz's Babesia and Bartonella Treatment

Dr. Horowitz wisely believes that the illness caused by Bartonella has been minimized or ignored. If both Babesia and Bartonella are present along with Lyme, one treatment option is to use the following plan:

• Septra DS or Bactrim DS at one tablet two times a day. He has found that doubling this dosage to one tablet four times per day causes markedly high and unacceptable side effects, so he no longer recommends this dose. This medication also has Babesia-killing abilities.

• Combine Septra DS with Mepron and a "macrolide" antibiotic such as Zithromax, Ketek or Biaxin. The evidence for the killing ability of macrolides is largely limited to Zithromax, but due to similar killing properties, Dr. Horowitz feels most macrolides have a theoretic role in combination with Mepron.

- Another effective option for treating Babesia, Bartonella and Lyme would be the use of Malarone, Levaquin, Plaquenil and Doxycycline.

Dr. Horowitz's (Rarely Used) AggressiveTreatment

The options above are usually fully successful. In **very rare** instances, (perhaps once a year), he uses oral Clindamycin or Quinine.

- Clindamycin in 300 mg capsules, taken as two capsules three times a day.

- Quinine 325 mg capsules, two capsules three times a day.

Again, this option is rarely used because the other treatments above almost always work. Further, this treatment has annoying side effects like ringing ears, rashes, nausea, vomiting, etc. In published abstracts Dr. Horowitz has illustrated that Clindamycin and Quinine had an unacceptably high failure rate.

If this treatment option is used, Malarone is sometimes added in order to help control Babesia.

Babesia Treatment for the Dying Patient

Most American Babesia is generally not fatal. However, in rare cases a patient will require a traditional hospital that is able to perform a blood exchange transfusion. Articles discussing this option do not mention if anti-Babesia medications are also given with the transfusion. I am also not aware what types of Babesia patients receive this care. However, the following patients seem to be considered for a transfusion:

1) People who have 10% or more of their red blood cells filled with Babesia infection

2) Individuals with massive amounts of blood cells bursting

3) A person with a Babesia infection and who does not have a spleen to filter out the infected red blood cells[114]

Individual Babesia Treatments in Detail

Treatments, Medications and Herbs

Let's discuss the most important information about common therapies and medications that can be used to treat Babesia. Later in the book we will discuss a medication called nitazoxanide (Alinia) that *might possibly* be useful for killing Babesia since it kills many different parasites and infections. tafenoquine (Etaquine) also has a good safety record, low side effects and **completely kills Babesia microti parasites.** However, tafenoquine is not yet available in the United States.

The following are important treatments and medications for Babesia:

- **Hyperbaric Oxygen**
- **Mepron**
- **Zithromax**
- **Malarone**
- **Lariam**
- **Artemesinin and Artemisia's other derivatives**
- **Heparin**
- **Quinine**
- **Clindamycin**
- **Bactrim or Septra**
- **Antifungals**
- **Doxycycline**
- **Plaquenil**
- **Primaquine**
- **Cholestyramine**
- **Glucosamine**
- **Etaquine**
- **Alinia**

Hyperbaric Oxygen

Hyperbaric oxygen involves a person entering a chamber that provides high levels of oxygen under varying degrees of pressure. It is known to help with various wounds and very specific infections. Some feel it also aids in healing neurons. I am only aware of two studies using Hyperbaric oxygen or high-dose oxygen therapy in the treatment of malaria or Babesia.

In one study, malaria-infected mice were given 100% oxygen at 3 atmospheres. (An "atmosphere" is a measure of pressure equal to about 33 feet of water above you). The number of red blood cells were the same in the healthy mice as compared to the malaria-infected mice. However, the red blood cells with malaria were reduced in number by 55-60% when measured promptly following the high hyperbaric treatment.[115] It should be noted that 3 atmospheres is generally considered an aggressive oxygen treatment that could have possible side effects to a human.

In another study, malaria cultures were exposed to oxygen at 1%, 20% and 50% of the air in the culture. No differences were noted in malaria growth between these oxygen concentrations and other gas samples. While this testing did not use any increased pressure, due to the poverty of data about this topic, I am including it here for examination.[116]

My experience is that most patients using hyperbaric treatments are also taking medications designed to kill Babesia, so any "success" could be from the medication and not the oxygen treatment. Further, we are aware of patients closely monitored for the effects of hyperbaric oxygen upon their Babesia, and the Babesia was present following treatment. While this fact could be related to perhaps another tick bite following the end of treatment, (especially in tick epidemic areas), I am unaware of data or clear clinical experience showing Babesia actually killed by hyperbaric oxygen.

Unfortunately, tick-borne infections are grossly ignored by many hyperbaric oxygen treatment centers, including centers sitting in the middle of counties having massive numbers of infectious deer ticks. Many of these centers seem bizarrely prejudiced and anti-scientific in their thinking that tick infections are not killed by hyperbaric oxygen despite the absence of data about those same beliefs. Obviously, more research and more concern is needed to clearly answer the clinical question of whether or not hyperbaric oxygen kills Babesia.

Mepron (atovaquone)

Most practitioners consider Mepron a highly effective front-line Babesia treatment option. Its killing ability may be attributed to the inhibition of Babesia enzymes. Mepron is a highly fat-loving medication that is absorbed twice as rapidly in liquid form. This is why it is offered as a thick yellow liquid. Therefore, a tablet will only be absorbed one-half as well as the comparable liquid form. Additionally, **taking it with food approximately *doubles* the rate of absorption.**

Blood levels of Mepron increase readily with only 500 mg per day, and each subsequent increase offers a modest increase in blood level—though less than what would be expected. Doubling the dose does **not** double the blood level of the drug. Mepron does not appear to reach high levels in the brain, as one study showed brain fluid levels under 1% of total blood levels. Mepron remains in the body much longer than most medications. It takes about 1-4 days in the blood for the medication level to drop 50%. It is excreted from the body by the liver into the stool.

Mepron has been used in very young children, (e.g., children with HIV). Some clinicians recommend a dosing of 10-25 mg/kg/day. However, please review this dosing recommendation with your pediatrician or health care specialist. Adolescents are typically treated with adult doses of 750 mg per teaspoon (5 mls) twice daily, to be taken with food.

Mepron liquid is bright yellow and has a citrus flavor. It comes in bottles of 210 milliliters, and should never be frozen. Mepron costs $856.00 wholesale for 210 mls. If you are taking two teaspoons per day (10 mls per day), a 210 ml bottle will last twenty-one days. Add to this wholesale price 15-20% for small pharmacies offering personal service. A large chain pharmacy or super discount store may only add 10%, but you might have to wait in a long line or wait a day or two for your prescription to be filled.

Mepron Side Effects

- Headache
- Fever
- Insomnia
- Rash

- Cough
- Nausea
- Vomiting
- Diarrhea
- Anxiety
- Dizziness
- Itch
- Belly discomfort
- Constipation

Mepron Interactions

Rifampin and Mepron together result in a 50% reduction in Mepron levels and a significant reduction in Rifampin levels. Other medications may interact with Mepron, but they do not appear to have clinical significance.

Mepron Lab Abnormalities

- Excess amylase
- Low sodium levels
- Low glucose levels
- Increased liver enzyme levels
- High kidney labs (high BUN/creatinine)
- Anemia
- Low white infection cell number (a low WBC)
- Low neutrophil number

The labs above can easily be checked with a routine comprehensive metabolic blood test and a blood amylase level.

How Mepron Works

Mepron is similar to the human body's naturally produced CoQ10. CoQ10 is used to make all the "gasoline" or ATP of the body. Mepron appears to impact Babesia by undermining or inhibiting production of CoQ10, a substance that Babesia needs for its metabolism. Mepron might also undermine the synthesis of ATP in the body, also negatively affecting Babesia. Perhaps this is one reason why clinicians suggest avoiding the use of CoQ10 supplements while taking Mepron. They are concerned the CoQ10 might prevent Mepron from fully working to kill Babesia.

Mepron and Pregnancy

Pregnancy safety is unknown and Mepron is a Class C Drug (See Appendix A).

Mepron and Zithromax in Combination

Many experts in tick-borne infection treatment routinely use Mepron and Zithromax together. This combination is so common lets look more closely at this approach, since both time and money should be considered if you use this treatment.

In one study, the Mepron group received 750 mg twice a day along with azithromycin (Zithromax), at 250 mg per day for a total of a week. Other patients were given another malaria treatment, clindamycin 600 mg every 8 hours with quinine 650 mg every 8 hours for a week. Only 15% who took both Mepron and Zithromax reported any side effects, the most common being diarrhea and rash. On the other hand, a full **72% of the clindamycin/quinine group reported side effects, with the most common being ear ringing, diarrhea and decreased hearing.** Side effects were sometimes slow to resolve and typically stopped after 2-5 months. The authors suggested that all Babesia microti was killed based upon microscope examination of blood and DNA blood testing. They concluded that Mepron with Zithromax was an effective treatment for Babesia with low side effects.[117,118]

Zithromax (azithromycin)

Zithromax is in a class of antibiotics called Macrolides. (Biaxin is another macrolide which is much more affordable). Some clinicians believe any macrolide like Biaxin or Ketek may augment Mepron. But so far the only clear research performed on this class of medications is that Zithromax, when taken with Mepron, has been found to help kill Babesia. It appears to work by disrupting protein synthesis.

Zithromax Side Effects

- Diarrhea
- Headache
- Nausea
- Abdominal pain
- Vomiting

Rare Serious Zithromax Side Effects

- Renal failure
- Agitation
- Heart risks–QTc EKG changes, torsade de points, etc.
- Jaundice (yellow palms, eyes and skin from liver injury)
- Seizures
- Deafness
- Pancreatic injury
- A profound entensive shedding rash
- Liver damage
- A fall in infection-fighting white blood cells (WBC's fall)[119]

Zithromax Drug Interactions

Since Zithromax can cause diarrhea, it may cause other medications to be absorbed at a lower rate since some medication is lost in rapidly moving stool. In terms of liver interactions,

Zithromax has some small interactions with drugs using the CYP3A4 liver enzyme system. Some think it is possible that Zithromax can impact levels of the following medications: ergot alkaloids, alfentanil, tacrolimus, bromocriptine, carbamazepine, cyclosporine, digoxin, disopyramide and triazolam. It is important to note that nelfinavir might increase Zithromax blood levels.

Available Forms of Zithromax

The suspension liquid form has a markedly better absorption rate, i.e., over 45% more is absorbed if taken with food.

- Tablets are available in 250 mg, 500 mg and 600 mg strengths.

- Injection form is 500 mg per shot into the muscle.

- Various liquid forms offer 100 mg, 200 mg or 1000 mg doses.

Not every pharmacy offers these options and some options may come in and out of production.[120]

Dosing of Zithromax

Currently I am unaware of dosing amounts approved for infant use. While the CDC suggests 10 mg/kg/day for 5 days for various infections, it does not offer any clear dosing for

Babesia. Discuss treatment options with your treating physician, but understand that studies using Zithromax and Mepron together for Babesia in infants or even children **do not exist** as of this printing. No one can guarantee the safety and effectiveness of the dose and duration of either Zithromax (or Mepron) for Babesia based upon our current, limited studies.

Zithromax and Pregnancy

Pregnancy Category B drug (See Appendix A).

Malarone: a Malaria Medication with Fewer Side-Effects

Over the years, malaria has developed antibiotic resistance to different treatments. Malarone is a newer medication marketed as a preventive treatment in areas of the world having chloroquine-resistant malaria. Malarone appears to be quite effective in *preventing* malaria.

Malarone is actually a combination of two medications, atovaquone (Mepron) and proguanil. It appears to work by preventing malaria's ability to make its own DNA. Malarone's main appeal is that it has fewer side effects than other malaria medications. Its drawback is its lower ability to kill malaria, and it is more expensive then other drugs used to kill both malaria and Babesia.

Malarone has been available in Denmark since 1998 and was approved for use in the United States in 2000. Malarone was designed to treat malaria already resistant to other treatments. Some believe it is unable to treat severe and advanced forms of malaria, such as neurological malaria, or fluid in the lungs or kidney failure due to the malaria. Further, in patients who only received Malarone for malaria, it was common for them to later relapse. Like Mepron, Malarone should be taken with fatty food or a milk-containing beverage.

Malarone 250 mg tablets cost $143.00 wholesale for 24 tablets. If you are only using one a day to merely keep Babesia moderately controlled, this supply can last nearly a month. If you are trying to be aggressive and take 750 mg twice a day, 24 tablets will last only six days. Add to this wholesale price 15-20% for small pharmacies offering personal service. Keep in mind larger chain pharmacies may charge less but make you wait longer.

Malarone Dosage

The dosing for malaria *prevention* is much lower than for the *treatment* of malaria. The adult dose for malaria prevention is one tablet per day. One tablet has only 250 mg of atovaquone (Mepron) and 100 mg of proguanil. The child dose for malaria prevention is one pediatric tablet (62.5 atovaquone/25 mg proguanil) for children of 11-20 kilograms. It is twice this dose for 21-30 kilogram children. Children weighing 31-40 kilograms take three pediatric tablets, and youths weighing 40 kilograms or more should take an adult dose.

Adults with active malaria take 1000 mg. This equals a tablet form of 1000 mg of atovaquone (Mepron) and 400 mg of proguanil each day as a single large dose.

Children with active malaria are dosed based on their weight. Infants weighing 5-8 kilograms take two pediatric tablets for three days. Children weighing 11-20 kilograms take one adult tablet for three days, while children weighing 31-40 kilograms take three adult tablets for three days. The exact dosing for the treatment of Babesia should be discussed further with your physician. The tablets can be crushed and mixed with food or milk to increase absorption levels and also facilitate their delivery to children.

Malarone Safety: Tablet Identification

- Adult Malarone tablets are pink and have "GX CM3" on one side.

- Child Malarone tablets are pink and have "GX CG7" on one side.

Pharmacists are trained to read these codes, but if you ever wonder if you have the correct prescription, you can read off these numbers to confirm your Malarone is the correct strength.

Common Malarone Side Effects

• Vomiting—if this occurs the medication may be expelled in the vomit. Therefore, anti-vomiting medications should be used, and a much lower starting dose should be considered.

• Diarrhea—if this occurs the medication may be moved too quickly through the gut and absorption may be reduced. Consult your physician if this occurs.

• Abdominal pain

• Nausea

• Headache

• Fever

• Muscle ache

• Belly pain

• Asthenia (loss of strength, weakness)

• Decreased appetite

• Cough

• Flu symptoms

• Upper respiratory infection

• Indigestion

• Dizziness

• Back pain

• Rash

- Sun sensitivity causing a rash
- Stomach irritation
- Angioedema (allergic swelling)
- Itching
- Dreaming
- Insomnia
- Mouth ulcers
- Reversible hair loss (which can also be caused by abnormal hormones or indoor mold exposure)
- Scaling skin on the soles of the feet and/or palms of hands

Rare Serious Malarone Side Effects

- Anaphylaxis or shock can occur, making breathing very difficult and requiring immediate emergency medical care.
- Erythema multiforme – a dangerous rash usually caused by an immune response to a drug or an infection.
- Stevens-Johnson syndrome – massive rash with full-body peeling of dead skin.
- Seizures
- Psychosis with hallucinations or delusions

Malarone Blood Test Changes

ALT and AST blood levels occasionally may be increased while using this medication. It is unknown if liver-protectant nutrients would prevent these changes. Once Malarone is discontinued, it may be a month or two before levels return to normal. It is also unclear to me if this process is due to the malaria or the medication.

Pre-existing Kidney Disease and Malarone Treatment

Patients with severe kidney disease need to be treated with extreme caution. Specifically, if their creatinine clearance is less than 30 ml/minute, Malarone should not be considered unless a clear infection and all other agents have failed or are not functional. Little research exists on Malarone use in Babesia patients with severe kidney disease. Individuals with mild or moderate kidney disease, e.g., creatinine clearance of 30-80 ml/minute can probably be treated with Malarone. Consider consulting either a urologist or a physician with expertise in kidney disease.

Fewer neuropsychiatric adverse experiences occurred in subjects who received Malarone than those receiving Lariam (mefloquine). Gastrointestinal adverse experiences are not routine. Compared with similar medications, Malarone has far fewer side effects.

Malarone Interactions with Other Medications

When Malarone is combined with tetracycline, the Malarone blood levels appear to be reduced about 40%. Since anti-nausea and anti-vomiting medications are sometimes needed when taking Malarone, please note the anti-nausea medication metoclopramide can lower the useful dose of Malarone. This anti-nausea medication should not be your physician's first choice when you are taking Malarone. Rifampin or Rifabutin both lower Malarone levels. **Rifampin cuts Malarone levels approximately in half.** Rifabutin drops Malarone levels by one-third. In light of these significant interactions, the use of these medications together is not recommended.

Proguanil is the second medication in Malarone, and it is metabolized in the liver by specific enzymes, the 2C19, 1A2 and 3A4 enzymes. It is unknown if it interacts with other medications which may also use these enzymes. Some clinicians feel Proguanil is only weakly interactive with other medications.

Pregnancy and Malarone

Malarone is not licensed for pregnant women and is a pregnancy category C medication. (See Appendix A).

Lariam

Lariam is the brand name for mefloquine. I think one of its main benefits is cost. Forms of artemesinin and Lariam are often combined to offer a cost effective combination malaria treatment. Specifically, Lariam 250 mg tablets cost about $310 retail per 25 tablets, or about $70.00 retail for five tablets. Since most people only take one tablet every 5-7 days, patients without insurance coverage only have to pay for a mere four to six tablets **per month.**

Lariam has had some bad publicity due to psychiatric side effects and occasional seizures. Despite these possible effects, I use it in individuals who have a limited income. It does have the capacity to cause almost any psychiatric problem, **so I begin with about one-eighth of a tablet.** Why? Because you can always increase the dose, and increase it fairly quickly, but once you take a dose that is too high, and causes side effects, it is hard to reverse the uncomfortable sensations. If this dose causes no allergic reactions or other side effects, I increase the Lariam by one-quarter tab units until it is obvious that the person can handle an entire tablet.

Sometimes patients experience some anxiety, depression or insomnia on Lariam, and yet choose to remain on their Lariam by taking psychiatric medications to treat their anxiety, depression or insomnia. I feel if this approach is attempted, that the Lariam should be discontinued first, and then the psychiatric medications stabilized, before a second trial of Lariam is tried. I also feel this should only be done by a psychiatrist who is at least briefly checking your emotional state weekly. These are highly personal decisions to be made in close consultation with your treating physician. **But be clear that continuing or increasing Lariam with any psychiatric symptom represents a risk.**

Newer package instructions suggest that some patients should *not* be given Lariam if they have any of the following conditions:

- Recent seizures
- Major depression
- Generalized anxiety or panic attacks
- Any type of thought disorder (hallucinations, paranoid behaviors, new confusion)
- Liver illness
- Significant agitation
- Heart block
- A pulse under 60 beats per minute
- A prolonged QT Interval on a routine EKG
- A previous adverse reaction to quinine and quinidine

If a person has any of the above conditions, it is usually best that they not be given Lariam. If Lariam must be used, the reasoning must be exceptionally clear and documented since treatment for Babesia and other tick-borne infections have innumerable people willing to second-guess any and all aspects of your medical treatment.

Lariam Side Effects

- Personality changes
- Tremor
- Trouble walking
- Mood abnormalities
- Panic attacks
- Confusion
- Suicidal thoughts
- Chest pain
- Swelling
- Indigestion
- Nausea or vomiting
- Blurred or loss of vision
- Disturbed color vision
- Dizziness
- Double vision
- Hearing trouble, ringing or buzzing sounds in ears
- Bladder control problems
- Light sensitivity
- A severe headache
- Trouble breathing

- Diarrhea
- Loss of appetite
- Rash
- Trouble sleeping
- Fatigue
- Loss of hair
- Flushing
- Heartburn or indigestion
- Skin rashes—mild or severe

Lariam and Pregnancy

Lariam should only be used if no other options are possible. It is rated as a Pregnancy category C medication. (See Appendix A).

Breastfeeding with Lariam

Lariam passes into breast milk. Yet it is generally believed that the small amounts in breast milk will not kill malaria. Therefore, based on the similarities between malaria and Babesia, it is unlikely the amount in the milk would kill any Babesia in an infant. If you have Babesia, you might want to stop your Lariam, since your infant could have side effects even from the low dose of Lariam in your breast milk. Some patients choose another medication while breastfeeding. Little research exists on the effects of Lariam on young infants.

Lariam and Older Adults

There is little information about the use of Lariam in the elderly. The elderly are often more sensitive to adverse effects of medications, including Lariam. So initial low dosing is probably wise in these individuals.

Lariam Drug Interactions

Interactions can be minimal or serious. Here are some interactions that are important. If you are going to use Lariam, let your doctor know you are taking the following medicines:

- Seizure medications such as carbamazepine, phenytoin or valproic acid may require a dose adjustment. (Lariam may also directly increase seizure risk).

- Chloroquine with Lariam can increase the chance of seizures.

- Halofantrine with Lariam may cause serious heart problems.

- Quinidine or Quinine with Lariam may cause heart reactions and also an increased risk of seizures.

- Penicillamine

- Live bacterial vaccines

- Beta-blockers that slow the heart rate

- QT prolonging agents, e.g., various anti-psychotics such as ziprasidone. For this reason it might be wise to order an EKG before Lariam use, and after the initial dose, to check the QT interval. Of course, if money is highly limited, some patients might prefer not to have this repeated.

- Typhoid vaccine

Lariam Instructions

Lariam or mefloquine is best taken with a full glass of water, with food, or crushed and taken with water, milk, or fruit juice.

Child Dosing with Lariam

Commonly, Babesia dosing is similar to that used for malaria, but often for a longer duration. Expert Babesia physicians have different recommendations, some of which we have already discussed, and some other sample dose options are outlined below.

- Children weighing 12 to 20 pounds should receive 5 mg of Lariam per kg of body weight each week.

- Children weighing 21 to 43 pounds take 62.5 mg or one-quarter of a tablet per week.

- Children weighing 44 to 66 pounds take 125 mg or one-half tablet per week.

• Children weighing 67 to 99 pounds take 187.5 mg or three-quarters of a tablet per week.

Malaria Dosing and Babesia Dosing

The malaria life cycle and the malaria organism is similar to those found in Babesia. However we cannot assume they should be treated in the same manner. Further, since there is not one type of Babesia, but many Babesia species that infect humans, treatments will differ depending on the species and how many months, years or decades it was missed.

While I have discussed Lariam risks in Babesia treatment, the fact is many patients with malaria have been able to tolerate high dose Lariam without any problems. Perhaps this means many people can tolerate Lariam better then we might think.

For example, aggressive treatment of malaria uses very high Lariam doses, e.g., in adults this can range from 750 mg to 1250 mg in **one day** (3-5 tablets) with an additional 500 mg or the optimal weight-based amount later in the **same day**! This means 5-7 tablets in the very first day of active malaria treatment.

For aggressive child malaria dosing, children usually are given 10 mg per pound in a divided dose, with one-half given in the morning, and the rest later in the day to lower side effects.

Preventing Accidents

Lariam can make you light-headed or impair your vision. Therefore, if you have either side effect, do not drive, use dangerous machines or use a ladder. It is better to simply avoid all heights. Call your physician to have your dose adjusted if your level of alertness, thinking or vision changes. Never drive if you are "foggy."

Artemisia's Amazing Ability
to Kill Red Blood Cell Infections and Cancer

As you may recall malaria and Babesia have many similarities. Not only do they look moderately similar as parasites of red blood cells, but also, as you have seen above, the same medications are used to treat both. Therefore, since Artemisia herbal medicines are so incredibly powerful and fast at killing malaria, and since Artemisia products are already used by patients to treat Babesia, we should examine this herbal option closely. Particularly, since the information that follows is **not available in any source except my new Artemisia book.** (Available from Amazon.com as a soft-cover or as an immediate download E-book from www.HopeAcademic.com).

Artemisia is a revolutionary herb that is the source for many new medications such as artemisinin. The derivatives of this herb are so important that the World Health

Organization and many other medical agencies recommend that approximately 400 million yearly malaria victims should receive this as their malaria treatment.[121,122]

Artemisia medicines are stunningly important. This Chinese herb is the first-line treatment for a massive medical illness—malaria. This information is stunning and historic. Allopathic physicians do not prescribe herbs, and the FDA does not even allow physicians to prescribe herbs or make specific health claims for any of them.

Finally, Artemisia and its derivatives appear to have both red blood cell parasite and cancer-killing properties. Specifically, infected cells or cancers absorb Artemisia medicines and then this herbal medicine creates powerful sparks or free radicals to kill the infected red blood cell or cancer cell from the inside–like a firecracker inside a paper milk carton.

Artemisia medicines seem to kill some types of cancers more effectively than others. For example, the most beneficial effects of this herb seem to be against leukemia, colon cancer, and melanoma. It also appears to have the ability to kill breast cancer, ovarian cancer, prostate cancer, brain cancer, some kidney cancers and many other cancers.[123-125]

Artemisia and Infections

Artemisia annua is known in the United States as "Sweet

Wormwood," "Sweet Annie" or "Annual Wormwood." It is often sold in the United States as artemisinin. It is native to many Asian countries, including China, where it is known as *Qinghao* or *Qinghaosu*.

Artemisia has been used medically for over 2,000 years, and it is mentioned in both the *Recipes For 52 Kinds Of Diseases* found in 168 B.C., and in the *Handbook of Prescriptions for Emergency Treatments*, written in 340 A.D. In 1596, artemisinin was named as a treatment for malaria by Li Shizhen. The major active ingredient was isolated in China in 1972.[126-128]

Currently various types of Artemisia annua seeds have been modified to grow all over the world. The herb may be found in Argentina, Bulgaria, France, Hungary, Romania, Italy, Spain, Africa, and the United States.[129]

A Boy's Miraculous Artemisinin Experience

Artemisinin is a common derivative of Artemisia and some patients use it against red blood cell parasites such as American Babesia and malaria throughout the world. Both live inside of red blood cells, and both appear to be killed by artemisinin. For little Xu Weifeng, artemisinin saved his life from malaria.

He nearly died from a raging fever when he was six years old. He lay upon a cot in a mountain hut surrounded by his parents, destined to become one more unknown victim of malaria.

"Every day the fevers began around four in the afternoon, and for the next ten hours I would not know if I was dreaming or dying," he recalled. Eventually a Chinese doctor gave him artemisinin and Xu quickly recovered. His artemisinin cure is now being hailed as a lifesaver for millions.[130]

Artemisia products have been used to treat over a million malaria patients. They are currently considered by the World Health Organization to be top treatments for malaria when used in combination with traditional long-acting malaria medications.[131] This is exactly the way many Babesia experts use Artemisia—in combination with a longer acting blood parasite medication such as those mentioned in previous sections.

It is also a malaria treatment researched by the United States military, perhaps due to the malaria exposure of American soldiers in Vietnam. It is already being grown by the United States Army in the state of Wisconsin, possibly for use by troops in Iraq and Afghanistan.

While it is grown throughout the world, one main growing region is a remote mountain range in central China, where farmers are now trying to satisfy the world's sudden demand. The Beijing Government is promoting mass cultivation of Artemisia, and the World Health Organization (WHO) plan to purchase about 100 million doses of the drug derived from this herb grown in China.

Mr. Xu, now 26 and fully recovered, is one of the local farmers converting entire valleys into shoulder-high Artemisia. As far as you can see, hillsides are covered with a sea of these lush green ferns. "In this region at least, there is no more malaria," Mr. Xu said.

The commercial development of Artemisia actually began when Vietnam asked China for help with their growing malaria problem in 1967. Beijing consulted an ancient medical text that included "qinghao," the Chinese word for artemisinin. A scholar named Ge Hong (281-340 AD) recommended "a handful of qing-hao in two pints of water" for illnesses that appear to be malaria.[132]

At present, not enough sweet wormwood is available or affordable to poorer countries like Africa. Part of this sudden shortage is the open endorsement of Artemisia products to fight malaria by major organizations such as the World

Health Organization (WHO) and the United Nations Children's Fund (UNICEF).[133-135]

The shortage has dramatically affected the cost of artemisinin, which has raised the price from $115 per pound to $455 per pound within a span of only 1-2 years.

Therefore, it has become unaffordable for full and effective dosing in economically disadvantaged countries. Because of this, the Gates foundation and medical companies are producing a bio-identical version of an Artemisia medication that uses single-celled bacteria to make an active form of Artemisia, (artemisinic acid). According to *Nature*, the production of artemisinic acid is already being grown in special yeast.[136,137]

It is expected to take five years to accomplish this process and set up a manufacturing process large enough to lower prices significantly. By then it is also hoped that the FDA and other European regulatory bodies will approve the herb. Currently in the United States it is considered a food item, so most medical insurance will not cover its cost.[138,139]

The mechanism that makes Artemisia useful in killing Babesia, malaria, and cancer, appears to be the same. Babesia and malaria parasites cannot eliminate iron within red blood cells, and many cancer cells collect iron. In all three uses, when artemisinin comes into contact with iron, a chemical reaction ensues which spawns free radicals.[140]

Handling Relapse Issues
with Malaria and Babesia

We know from malaria treatment that relapse rates drop if Artemisia medicines are used for longer periods and when another traditional malaria medication is added, e.g., Lariam. This is why some Babesia experts combine Artemisia products with long-acting synthetic medications. This combined Artemisia and synthetic medication approach is the new standard of care in treating malaria in Asia and Africa.

Another option is to add other pharmaceutical herbs to the Artemisia herb. In China, herbs are commonly added to other herbs to help the "master herb" work more effectively and to reduce resistance in which the herb loses its effectiveness.

For example, Dr. Zhang adds to his Artemisia, *allitridi*, the **stable** precursor to Allicin that causes garlic odor that is present in effective forms. (Chlorophyll reduces this odor). He also adds coptis (umbellatine), and HH (dodecane carboaldehyde and 3-oxo), which are broad infection killers that like Allicin are small enough to penetrate into the brain. Allicin, coptis, HH and his R-5081 formula can be added to kill Lyme.[141] Others are looking at adding the herb *curcumin* to artemisinin, which shows some preliminary possible effectiveness against Babesia.[142]

Forms of Artemisinin

Currently, there are a handful of common Artemisia products. They have very different properties, so lets discuss their basics to enable you to make smart decisions about medicines derived from Artemisia. Perhaps the most popular derivative of Artemisia in the United States is artemisinin, so lets start with this one.[143,144] Here is a brief look at the core practical facts of artemisinin.

Artemisinin

Artemisinin was the first medicine derived from the Artemisia plant. Now it is one of the key active parent compounds used to make other synthetic forms. Artemisinin has a modest duration within the body. Approximately one-third is absorbed into the bloodstream when taken orally. Artemisinin easily crosses the intestinal wall into the blood, and this ability does not change with repeated dosing.[145,146] Its potency within the body is low. For example, by contrast, artesunate is 4 to 5 times more active in the body than artemisinin.[147]

Artemisinin is considered quite safe, and yet is able to cross the blood-brain barrier. Since artemisinin can enter the brain, it is effective for cerebral forms of malaria. In one study, malaria fevers ended in 72 hours, and it also clearly removed malaria parasites. However, there was a relapse rate of 21% when treatment duration lasted only three days. Artemisinin is not a new herb with little research or clinical use. It has been extensively researched for malaria, and has been used on over a million patients, mostly in China and Vietnam.

One major concern with artemisinin is that it induces its own removal. Amazingly, **after only 5 days, the blood levels fall to one-fifth of the dose administered on day one.**[148] Most practitioners are unaware that therapeutic blood levels drop this rapidly (due to auto-induction of liver enzymes). This ramping up of artemisinin removal enzymes begins just two hours after the very first dose.[149] However, despite this induction of the liver that removes artemisinin very rapidly, **the blood level of the active metabolite, dihydroartemisinin, increases with repeated treatment.**[150]

Artemisinin often cures malaria with a nominal dose of 250 mg per day. In one study, after a week of treatment, all patient blood was clear of malaria parasites and none had fevers. It appeared the malaria was largely killed within the first three days.[151] However, this study raises two issues, what is the "ideal dose" and what is a "cure." First, the dosing recommended by the World Health Organization for a 60-kg adult is **1200 mg on the first day, followed by 600 mg on the following day.**[152]

Second, many studies claim 100% elimination of malaria within 3-7 days, but this is inaccurate. When any brief follow-up is conducted, (months or seasons after treatment), we find approximately 8-39% relapse with a return of the patient's malaria.[153-156]

Dihydroartemisinin

The majority of the herbal medicine varieties derived from Artemisia end up as dihydroartemisinin, which is the herb's active metabolite. This means that most Artemisia medicines become dihydroartemisinin, which is the active ingredient that kills malaria and presumably Babesia.

Dihydroartemisinin was prescribed to men and women at a dose of 2 or 4 mg/kg for malaria, and it performed well. Both doses had minimal side effects and both were rapidly absorbed from the intestines. There was no significant difference between men and women in absorption or blood levels.[157] In 53 patients in another study, a total daily dose of 480 mg in adults every day for a week showed a malaria cure rate of 90%.[158]

Artemether

This form is able to pass through fat in the body. It has the longest duration, but is also the most toxic form in high dosages–levels that are rarely necessary. This form is available overseas in both oral and injectable forms. Grapefruit juice blocks the liver metabolism of this medication and allows it to last longer.[159]

The biggest advantage of artemether is that it can cross the blood-brain barrier. This synthetic form has been used in thousands of patients. If it is used for only 3-5 days, malaria relapses are common. Artemether is widely used for acute malaria. The oral form of artemether is poorly absorbed through the intestines as compared to artesunate.[160]

Artesunate

This is a highly respected form of Artemisia that is the most active and the least toxic. It is also water-soluble. This form has a very short duration within the body and is 4 to 5 times more active in the body than artemisinin.[161] Artesunate is a synthetic form that has been used in thousands of patients. When taken for only 3-5 days, relapses are common.

This form is available overseas in both oral and injectable doses. In a comparison of oral artesunate and artemether, oral artesunate administration resulted in significantly higher blood activity time and better malarial killing. Further, oral blood levels of artemether were significantly lower than found with oral artesunate.[162]

Sample studies of artesunate have often used 50-250 mg tablets. Daily doses have ranged from 600 to 1200 mg per day with or without a second synthetic antimalaria agent, e.g., Lariam.[163]

One study of children with malaria given injectable artesunate showed it rapidly entered the bloodstream, with the maximum concentration of dihydroartemisinin (the main antimalarial metabolite), being achieved in under an hour in most children's blood. There were no major adverse events attributable to artesunate in the study. These results support using injectable artesunate in children with severe malaria.[164] The application of this study to the treatment of Babesia is currently unknown.

Very little is known about the peak concentration and duration of artesunate in the body. A dose of 150 mg of artesunate was fed **orally** to lab rats with the following results:[165]

- Blood levels of artesunate peaked within only 5 minutes.

- Blood levels of dihydroartemisinin peaked within 37 minutes.

In another study, when 120 mg of artesunate was administered to patients **intravenously,** the duration of the Artemisia derivatives were again found to be amazingly short.

- Half of the artesunate was gone from the body within 3.5 minutes.

- Half of the active metabolite, dihydroartemisinin, was gone within 34 minutes.[166-168]

Therefore, artesunate is very rapidly converted into dihydro-artemisinin by stomach acid. The fact that artesunate reaches an early peak in the stomach within minutes of dosing is amazing.[169] Further, oral artesunate produces high levels of dihydroartemisinin, the potent functional metabolite, very quickly. However these levels do not last long, and so oral artesunate is recommended for *repeated* dosing throughout the day.

Arteether

This medication is available in an injectable form and is metabolized slowly. It also has a longer duration in the body as compared to other artemisinin derivatives. Only 5% is converted to dihydroartemisinin. Arteether has an alpha and a beta part. The alpha part causes a rapid and significant blood level, and the beta part converts minimally and slowly to dihydroartemisinin and lasts longer in the body.[170,171]

Dr. Zhang's "Artemisinin"

Dr. Zhang studied Chinese medicine for twenty years mastering Chinese herbal medicine. He then received fellowships to study traditional Western medicine at Harvard and in Japan. He has the ability to make very complex Chinese herbal medicine understandable. In his new book, *Lyme*

Disease and Modern Chinese Medicine, he discusses Babesia treatments. He reports success killing Babesia with a series of herbs from Hepapro, a company that makes a form of Artemisia called *Artemisia anomala S. Moore.*[172]

Actually, Artemisia anomala S. Moore has no ability to kill malaria or Babesia and was an accidental mislabeling. I have been told the new bottles have corrected labels with the name **Artemisia annae L** on the label. These capsules are actually **artesunate.**

Based upon decades of experience, Dr. Zhang has found that the synthetic and potent **artesunate is much more effective in killing malaria and Babesia.** His Artemisia capsules also have two other additional herbs to improve the effectiveness of the artesunate.[173]

His herbs can be ordered from:

> Hepapro
> P.O. Box 7442
> Laguna Niguel, CA 92607-7442
> Phone 888-788-4372 or Fax 949-363-7715

Over twenty forms of natural and synthetic Artemisia exist. However, in an effort to keep this book functional, we are only discussing the most common forms.

Compounded Artemisia: Suppositories

If you have a raw and painful stomach, one option is the use of Artemisia in a suppository. In one study, artesunic acid was prescribed as an intense treatment over one day's duration by inserting 200 mg suppositories every 6-8 hours into the rectum.[174]

Artemisinin Transdermal Cream

Transdermal forms show good potential. Artemisia in the form of artemether, dihydroartemisinin, artelinic acid, and artemisinin has been used in transdermal gels with good results. Complete absorption of dihydroartemisinin through the skin appears to occur within 5 minutes following application.

In general, the transdermal malaria **preventive** dosing is about **half the curative dose** for infected patients. Peak blood levels appear to be achieved between 30 minutes to 4 hours after application. Since most American compounding pharmacists can put most medications into a wide range of transdermal creams or gels, this option might be possible in the future.[175-177]

Artemisinin and Natural Vitamin A

The addition of vitamin A increases the effectiveness of artemisinin against malaria, and possibly against Babesia. The presence of vitamin A increases the killing power of artemisinin approximately 3 or 4 times. It is unknown what is the optimal dose of natural vitamin A. Pregnant women are told never to take over 4,000 International Units (IU) and men are told not to exceed more than 5,000 IU's a day. If you want a higher dose then you should get a consult with a progressive nutritionist. Synthetic forms of vitamin A such as Accutane, can cause fetal abnormalities if pregnant.[178,179] Further, the use of *cholestyramine* or *Welchol* to bind Lyme or mold biotoxins will also bind fat-soluble vitamins like vitamin A, in addition to the other fat-soluble vitamins D, E and K and lower their levels.

Artemisia Products and Cancer: A Brief Word

In addition to their anti-parasitic agents. Some research shows they have anti-cancer ability.[180-182]

Important possible beneficial effects of this herb seem to be against leukemia,[183-186] colon cancer, melanoma,[187-189] breast cancer,[190,191] ovarian cancer, prostate cancer,[192] brain cancer[193] and kidney cancer. Other cancers that appear to show some possible useful Artemisia benefits[194-198] include:

Cervical cancer[199,200]

Liver cancer[201,202]

Kaposi's Sarcoma[203]

Astrocytoma Cancer[204]

Fibrosarcoma Tumors[205,206]

Oral Squamous Cell Carcinoma[207]

Ovarian Cancer[208,209]

Small-Cell Lung Cancer[210,211]

Stomach Cancer[212]

In one laboratory study, resistant breast cancer cells had a high propensity for accumulating iron. When these iron-loaded cells were treated with artemisinin, they had a 75% cancer cell die-off within only 8 hours, and nearly a 100% die-off within 24 hours. On the other hand, normal cells not heavy with iron, remained virtually unharmed by artemisinin.[213-218]

Artemisinin and Low Body Iron

If we apply iron cancer information to killing malaria and Babesia, we gain even more information on Artemisia's mechanisms. First, many children and menstruating women have low iron levels. And sometimes these low iron levels do not show up in very basic labs. If you are found to have low iron or actual anemia, consider taking iron if taking Artemisia. If you only take iron for half of a week, we know from one study that Artemisia may not work as well with only **"fair"** supplementation.[219]

If your iron is low or your lab shows anemia, take aggressive dosing. If you are a women with periods lasting over six days per month, consult your physician to address possible estrogen dominance, which is a problem commonly missed. Low progesterone combined with higher estrogen levels causes poor blood vessel clamping, fibrocystic breasts and fibroids.[220]

Many iron products are available, but it appears that the one with the highest absorption rate, lowest side effects and which is the most effective to use with Artemisia is ferrous heme (Fe+2).[221,222] This special iron combines with all common forms of Artemisia to create reactions that kill malaria and Babesia.[223-225]

Therefore, if you are going to use Artemisia, make sure you have enough iron in your body by first running a full iron lab panel. In addition, one should check **ferritin**, which is a good body iron marker, and **hemoglobin** and **transferrin.** These labs allow you to make certain you have enough iron to combine with an Artemisia product to kill Babesia. Your ferritin levels should be above 45. As a trend, when taking this powerful herbal medicine, it is perhaps best to be in the top half of normal blood iron levels.

Taking iron with vitamin C (such as Ester-C) will increase the absorption of the iron. Taking iron with orange juice appears to **double** iron absorption. Conversely, zinc, calcium and magnesium taken with iron will **decrease** its absorption. Tea decreases iron absorption by approximately 75%.

Increasing Free Radical Sparks Increases Artemisinin Killing Ability

Medications like miconazole and doxorubicin work by increasing free radicals. In the same manner, we find that artesunate is even more effective at killing malaria and probably Babesia, with free radicals promoted by iron. Malaria or Babesia in human red blood cells contains significant iron as part of their oxygen transport ability. Artemisia medicinal herbals kill parasites by using iron to generate free radicals. Artemisinin peroxides generate free radicals when exposed to iron. **Electron microscope images show malaria membranes treated with artemisinin are destroyed in ways typical of free radical killing.**[226]

Lowering Free Radicals or Wild Bullets: The Basics

When artemisinin and ferrous iron combinations are exposed to free radical **catchers** like NAC, glutathione, catalase, vitamin C and vitamin E, **less malaria is killed but other body tissues are protected.**[227-229]

One of the ways people become slowly ill and eventually die is due to years of free radical damage. The same free radicals used to fight malaria and Babesia, cause aging and organ damage over time. One might imagine these free radicals as being bullets in a fireplace. Human cells make energy in select areas of the cell that are like "fireplaces." But while the cell is making energy, some bullets shoot out of the cell furnaces, which we call "free radicals." They can damage a wide range of cell parts, just as a wild bullet can. The good news is that we can catch these free radical bullets. The body has built-in enzymes and nutrients to catch these destructive free radicals. Some individuals believe that body injury is occurring when iron and artemisinin "work" by making free radical bullets that kill malaria, Babesia or cancer.

Sample Anti-Oxidants and Babesia or Malaria

NAC is a natural chemical found in our liver. It is sold in virtually all health food stores and many pharmacies. It helps red blood cells **be less rigid from malaria or possibly Babesia so these red blood cells can move through the ultra-fine circulation.**[230] Malaria blocks the flow of red cells in tiny circulation tubes. Autopsies have proven this microcirculation obstruction exists in severe cases of malaria. Red blood cells become rigid and sticky and adhere to blood vessel linings, causing blockage. This can be very dangerous.

During a Babesia infection treated with Artemisia products, free radicals are harming Babesia according to Chinese physician Dr. Zhang, but I worry some free radicals also harm the body, and the blood vessel lining can become damaged. This is one reason anti-oxidants are good to add to your treatment, because they catch excess Artemisia free radicals. Artemisia free radicals help the immune system explode the parasite but are *not selective.*

We want a balance between two opposite extremes. **We want to promote free radical parasite killing, but we do not want our blood vessels or other organs injured by free radicals.** Two options might be of use in this scenario.

1) In severe malaria and probably severe Babesia, rigidity of red blood cells may increase organ damage and death. Since these rigid red cells seem to be caused by free radical damage to the red blood cell membrane, the anti-oxidant free radical "catchers" NAC, vitamin C and other anti-oxidants offer real promise in keeping blood cells both flexible and healthy.[231-233] Further, if we use iron in the top half of normal iron blood levels, together with Artmesia products, we will make free radicals inside the red blood cells to kill the parasites. But the free radical catchers like NAC will be around the red cells and prevent excess tissue damage from the iron-Artemisia free radicals. Further, if we use iron in the top half of normal iron blood levels, together with Artemisia products, we will make free radicals inside the red blood cells to kill the parasites. But the free radical catchers like NAC will be around the red cells and prevent excess tissue damage from the iron-Artemisia free radicals.

2) One interesting idea outside of Artemisia is the option to use a metal binder or chelator called *desferrioxamine,* which binds iron forms that produce free radicals. This drug has anti-parasite activity because iron is required for the reproduction of the parasite, and this medicine binds and removes iron.[234]

Side Effects of Artemisia

Most Artemisia studies report minimal side effects with these medicines. Well-documented clinical uses of Artemisia and its derivatives report these possible side effects below. However most patients have no trouble taking this medication.

- Skin tingling

- Reports of rare and transient heart block

- Possible heart palpitations

- Transient decreases in infection-fighting blood neutrophils

- Brief episodes of fever

- Possible liver or kidney effects based on an animal study

- Slight muscle aches after exertion due to low VEGF

- Nausea or vomiting

- Abdominal pain

- Diarrhea

- Low blood pressure

- Cardiac and intestinal toxicity has occurred in animals (usually with higher doses)

- Fetal loss within the first trimester[235-238]

Fatigue and low VEGF with Artemisia

In some of my other books, I discuss the studies of Dr. Shoemaker who has found that a low VEGF (vascular endothelial growth factor) can be caused by biotoxins from Lyme, mold, some lake algae and many other sources.

VEGF builds and opens capillaries and can be tested by a blood test with the best results from Quest labs, though not all Quest labs are up-to-date and able to offer it. Your local Quest lab can tell you if their processing lab does VEGF testing. If they do, it is usually covered by insurance.

Since Artemisia products lower VEGF, it is possible that these levels could become too low. In cancer treatment, the physicians like VEGF low because it means that the tumor is not getting a full blood supply. However, if one is not fighting cancer, a low VEGF can cause aches, foggy thinking and fatigue either during or after exertion. One way to treat it is to use cholestyramine at 3-4 packets per day to bind the biotoxin (like from Lyme disease), carefully remediate and remove any indoor mold, and use 9-10 omega 3 enteric coated fish oil capsules per day. The enteric coating prevents the fish oil from annoying your stomach.

Some individuals have VEGF levels that are too high. According to Dr. Shoemaker, this is a sign of VEGF malfunction. For example, if biotoxins are blocking the VEGF receptors, the blood level of VEGF could be very high because its receptors are blocked. We have found that he is right—both abnormally low and abnormally high VEGF levels are a sign of illness and commonly caused by biotoxins from Lyme, indoor mold and other biotoxins.[239,240]

Drug Interactions with Artemisinin

The liver has enzymes that help to remove medications and herbs. One important part of this system is the *cytochrome P450* enzyme system. These enzymes do the lion's share of medication removal. They easily remove some medications, while other medications inhibit these enzymes, driving up the drugs metabolized by them. Others induce these enzymes to increase in number so that blood levels of any drug specific for them will fall.

Artemisinin **induces CYP3A4.** Therefore, many of these enzymes are made and any medication metabolized by this enzyme will have a reduced blood level. When you have more enzymes of a certain class, you have less of the drug removed by that enzyme.[241]

Artemisinin also profoundly inhibits CYP1A2, so drugs that require this enzyme to be removed, will increase in the body.[242]

Finally, artemisinin creates many CYP2B6 enzymes. These enzymes cause the unusual drop in the blood level of artemisinin very rapidly after only 5 days. These increased 2B6's drop artemisinin levels to one-fifth as high as on day one. I would expect that other drugs metabolized by CYP2B6 might also be reduced.[243,244]

Ideally, your physician or other health care provider should have a list of medications metabolized by each of these three enzymes to see how any of your medications might interact with Artemisia. In today's reality, few health care practitioners have time to compare each of your medications to the form of Artemisia you may have purchased. Therefore, I would buy a drug interactions book or a drug handbook such as from USP (patient version) or Lexi-Comp's yearly medication handbook, so you can look up your own medications. This web site also offers large amounts of interaction data:

http://medicine.iupui.edu/flockhart/table.htm

However, the main section of this site might be too large for you. But at least look over their small table offering major drug interactions.

Can Malaria or Babesia Become Resistant to Artemisia and Its Derivatives?

Most of the world's malaria researchers feel that **any** form of malaria treatment can lose effectiveness over time. They fear that using weak Artemisia doses could allow some malaria to survive and become resistant. This is one reason they want to pair Artemisia derivatives with synthetic, longer-acting medications. As of this year, it appears that malaria resistance to artemisinin products has not yet occurred. However, some notice that effective dosing might need to be higher in some areas where Artemisia has been used for some time. (This is a complex issue, and this higher dosing issue could be attributed to many factors).

Below are two studies that show that it is possible, over time, to have resistance to Artemisia medicines. Resistance is the loss of effectiveness over time. So researchers sped up the process of testing for resistance by using mice infected with malaria.

In both studies they treated infected mice with an Artemisia medicine and then injected blood into another batch of mice and then repeated this process. After some time it did appear that more medication was required to have the same malaria-killing effect. Curiously, resistance seemed to come and go in these initial tests.

In these special texts, once every 7-10 days, red blood cells with parasites were passed on to the next group of mice, who were receiving the same doses of artemether, for 50 passages – 50 new groups of mice. Resistance development was slow but increased considerably over the final ten passages.

Importantly, resistance was unstable, since sensitivity reverted to near normal after five passages into healthy mice without Artemisia being used.

P. berghei (malaria) resistance was tested using artemether. In conclusion, the pace of resistance in P. berghei to repeated high doses of artemether is slow but can happen. In some study samples, the medication sensitivity can return to normal.[245,246]

Do Artemisinin Formulations Hurt the Human Brain? Examining Both Sides of the Issue

The active ingredient of artemisinin, dihydroartemisinin (DHA) is from *Artemesia annua L.* (sweet wormwood) but **not** from *Artemesia absinthium* (wormwood). This matters because traditional wormwood is known to have neurotoxins like *absinthe, thujone* and *isothujone*. Some poor studies and even poorer articles discuss the side effects of Artemisia and confuse sweet wormwood with wormwood, but they are not the same herb.[247]

The more important issue is whether artemisinin, DHA, artemether, artesunate or other sweet wormwood products can hurt the body, e.g., parts of the brain or hearing structures. As a trend, the Artemisia types suspected of these side effects are forms used in high doses, for a prolonged period of time and are synthetic versions of the herb. While I think this herb can be used safely, I do **not** think a person should take the herb without reading the facts on this issue. Individuals who say Artemisia products have "no side effects," are in error.

The World Health Organization is promoting the use of Artemisia-based medications for malaria treatment. The WHO is familiar with the studies that report various serious side effects, but they also are fully aware of the many malaria deaths each year. Therefore, this treatment is still being promoted for millions of malaria patients. It appears they do not feel this side effect is as serious as a small number of other researchers.

Perhaps the brain and hearing side effect worry began in 1994, when Breyer published results of his study using arteether at 20mg/kg/day in dogs for eight straight days. The dogs had significant neurological defects, and actual death occurred in five of six animals. Their neurological findings included walking problems, loss of pain sensation, and some brain function loss. In later follow up animal studies; Brewer noted many other findings, e.g., brain damage, EKG changes and seizure-like activity when using arteether or artemether.[248]

In a rat study using beta-arteether, (which is the longer acting arteether form), animals were given this herb in either long-acting sesame oil or a form rapidly removed. DHA is probably an active metabolite of arteether, so this was close-ly monitored.

The transport substance for the arteether mattered significant-ly in this study since **blood levels of arteether in sesame oil were 7.5-fold higher** in the final day of treatment. Brain tis-sue revealed some toxic changes in all animals. The extension of drug exposure time and constant detectable levels of arteether and dihydroartemisinin were more associated with severe neurotoxicity and less killing of malaria, while high levels and shorter exposure times resulted in greater malaria killing effects and milder toxicity.[249]

Scientists believe the side effects in this case are probably not due to low blood levels, but are more easily caused by intra-muscular shots that have slow absorption into the bloodstream and can result in a continuous and **prolonged high level of drug exposure.**[250]

Oral vs. Injected Forms of Artemisinin

In a comparison between injected artemether and injected arteether against common **oral** artemisinin forms, a number of important findings were noticed:

1) Brain toxicity occurred under **constant exposure** with either high dose injected, oil-based artemisinin deriva-

tives or constant oral intake.

2) **Oral** artemether, artesunate, and DHA had similar neuro-toxic effects, but with **no significant evidence of toxicity at doses below 200 mg/kg/day.**

3) The data also indicated that once or twice daily oral administration of artemether, artesunate and dihydroartemisinin is relatively safe when compared to intramuscular administration of the oil-based compounds. Oral doses spike and fall rapidly within hours of administration.[251]

Animal and Human Toxicity Studies

Some researchers feel the effects of artemisinin products vary considerably between rats, mice, dogs and humans. They feel that the application of animal studies to humans is dubious when millions of humans apparently have used these products with only trivial side effects. Others feel that 38 published animal studies and some initial human studies about Artemisia products clearly show a neurological risk and a hearing loss risk. These findings should not be ignored.[252]

Researchers affirm that we have used animals for drug testing for decades, and finding toxic side effects in artemisinin products cannot be ignored. Others feel that large mammals do fine with artemisinin medications and this is more of an issue with small mammals and not their larger human counterparts. This distinction is also true with mainstream pharmaceuticals.[253]

Human studies are exhibiting a wide range of results. While malaria itself can cause various brain injuries, individuals with **no malaria** who take arteether and who are not ill or on other medications, have had hearing damage.[254]

A few studies exist showing patients who did not have pre-existing ear disease, who while on artemether or artesunate in combination with other top malaria medications, subsequently developed ear disease.[255-258]

Other studies point to the use of artemisinin in millions of patients and the exceptionally rare findings of neurological damage with artesunate use.[259,260] Further, in individuals who died of severe malaria and who were treated with quinine and artemether, no unique neurological damage was found.[261]

One final piece of evidence is the effect of artemisinin products on brain tissue cultures. When living tissue in culture is exposed to Artemisia products, it appears that artemisinin and its products kill both neuronal and brain support cells (glial cells). Some cell tests show that significant cell toxicity is seen at dosages as low as 1-2 mg/kg of human body weight.[262-266]

In the *Toxicology Letter*, their conclusion on the issue of artemisinin brain toxicity was:

1) The prolonged presence of Artemisia products in the body due to the *slow release* of oil-based intramuscular injected formulations is the main cause of the observed toxicity in laboratory animals.

2) In contrast, oral intake of these compounds, which is by far the most common formulation used for treatment of malaria patients, results in rapid clearance of these drugs and is thus unlikely to cause any toxicity in human subjects.

3) The relatively high doses of artemisinin compounds used in animal studies cause toxic reactions in animals due to different effects in animals as opposed to humans.

4) Animals respond to different delivery routes in a way that promotes toxicity as compared to humans.[267,268]

Pregnancy Toxicity and Artemisia Derivatives

Moderate artesunate exposure to pregnant rabbits and rats had serious negative fetal effects including dramatic early embryo loss, rare heart and blood vessel abnormalities and many types of bone defects. These problems happened even in healthy animal mothers.

In order to radically reduce these risks, the artesunate cannot be greater than 5 mg/kg/day. In contrast, a human study of 700 pregnant women had markedly better results. No developmental effects were found in 100 first trimester mothers and 600 second and third trimester mothers treated with Artemisia derivatives, primarily artesunate. It is possible that rats and rabbits are more sensitive to Artemisia than humans.[269]

Conclusions to Toxicity Data

1) Millions of people have been exposed to artemisinin and other synthetic forms. Many have taken only 1-10 days of this herb. Nevertheless, if this group of herbal drugs easily damaged human brain stems or hearing systems, it would probably be obvious even with routine dosing and short durational use.

2) Animal cell cultures show that these herbal drugs can damage brainstem cells.

3) Massively high doses of any artemisinin drug causes mammal neurological damage.

4) Oil-based synthetically derived forms create a longer half-life, which results in **constant** and unremitting free radical effects on the brain.

5) Oral dosing allows for very fast and very high blood lev-

els followed by **the complete removal of the drug within hours,** thus allowing the brain a rest from free radicals.

6) High dosing which is continuous, e.g., IV or injected, that lasts three days or longer might be problematic.

7) I am unaware of studies that address the issue of liver enzyme induction in any form of Artemisia except artemisinin. This latter form falls quickly to low blood levels, while the active metabolite dihydroartemisinin increases.

8) The weight of the patient probably matters. Many studies are based on doses per kilogram. Since medication dosing is typically safest with an awareness of body weight, I do not believe this variable should be ignored.

9). In a study of artemether's toxicity, 68 patients were treated with artemether (and a malaria medicine lumefantrine) within the previous five years were matched with a control group of 68 people of the same age and gender. Both groups had the same functioning, with no auditory or brainstem toxicity found in the study group.[270]

10) Individuals with a genetic HLA pattern of 15-6-51 or 16-5-51 or other such patterns are individuals who do not remove Lyme's surface endotoxins or biotoxins naturally, and so they develop severe and extensive chemical reactions all over their body. (See Shoemaker,

Schaller and Schmidt. *Mold Warriors* for LabCorp HLA DR DQ test order codes with a significant explanation). Treating any tick-borne infection such as Babesia without awareness of this issue often leads to:

- Diverse and severe hormone abnormalities, e.g., marked alterations in MSH, VEGF, Free Testosterone, DHEA, Free T3 Thyroid and VIP

- Wide-ranging creation of abnormal inflammation chemicals

- Many types of autoimmunity

Dosing Recommendations: Oral Intermittent Dosing

While it is very clear that artemisinin and its related medications are exceptional medications to treat malaria, the correct dosing for Babesia or various cancers is unknown. Various communities, countries, clinicians and studies are using such a wide range of dosing that **authoritarian dosing suggestions are not possible.**

While we appreciate that many Chinese herbal experts are more aggressive than the suggestions below, we are simply trying to be careful. **Dosing artemisinin or its derivatives remains in a state of evolution. Yet this medicine has already been used in over 2 million patients with limited**

side effects. Therefore, this is *not* an experimental herb.

In high-quality studies it was found that synthetic artemether, when **orally** administered at a dose of 6 mg/kg **once** every 2-3 weeks, resulted in no drug-related adverse effects.[271]

In collaborative research between Chinese, European and African scientists, artemether showed no indication of neurotoxicity following repeated high doses of artemether when given **every 2 weeks** for up to 5 months. Note the long time span between doses.[272]

Artesunate taken at 4 mg/kg in one dose followed by a dose of Lariam appears to be safe. Yet this single dose combo leaves one-quarter to one-third of malaria alive. Therefore, single doses with Artemisia derivatives is probably a poor treatment option for both malaria and Babesia.[273]

Artesunate at 4 mg/kg/day combined with Lariam at 8 mg/kg/day administered orally once daily **for 3 days,** and dihydroartemisinin 40 mg with piperaquine at 320 mg once daily **for 3 days** were both successful at removing malaria, with no toxicity reported.[274]

Artemether given to dogs at a high daily dose of 135 mg/kg for 2 weeks did not cause severe side effects. This very high dose produced no hearing tissue damage or brain damage tissue signs when examined microscopically. Some dogs exhibited an increase in liver weight, and liver cell enlargement, and showed some changes within kidney cells.[275]

Nevertheless, high doses of injected Artemisia medicines can harm the brain stem in laboratory animals. This can happen to the brain of a dog in only three days following three oil-based injections or IV treatments with dihydroartemisinin, artemether and arteether in **doses exceeding about 6mg/kg/d intramuscular or intravenous for 3-5 days in a row with no break. The same damage occurs with a massive single injection of over 100 mg/kg.** Monkeys seem to require doses even higher for the same type of damage to occur. Rats appear to also require large dosing for brain damage to appear.

Some researchers believe that there is little reason to anticipate brain stem or hearing damage in humans if one is using artemether at 3-6mg/kg/day in a muscle-injected form or artesunate in rectal suppositories for three days.[276]

Dihydroartemisinin or artemether significantly inhibited neurons in small lab samples. This effect was prevented by exposure to the anti-oxidants superoxide dismutase, catalase, glutathione, L-cysteine, NAC (N-acetyl-L-cysteine) and ascorbic acid or Ester C (vitamin C). Glutathione prevents the neurotoxicity of artemether and dihydroartemisinin. Artemether depletes intracellular glutathione levels, whereas dihydroartemisinin had no effect. All of these anti-oxidants are available from my web site, at their published wholesale prices at: www.personalconsult.com.

Further, I have found many patients enjoy fruit-flavored **sublingual** glutathione. Sublingual pills or troche forms go right into the bloodstream–these are similar to nitroglycerine tablets, but these sublingual pills deliver glutathione rapidly into the bloodstream instead of nitroglycerine.

These glutathione prescription lozenges can be purchased in blueberry or tangerine flavors at Lionville Natural Pharmacy at 877-363-7474 or a prescription can be faxed to 610-363-5707. College Pharmacy in Colorado also has a pleasant-tasting tangerine glutathione sublingual tablet. The main number at College Pharmacy is 800-888-9358. Their fax number is 800-556-5893.[277,278]

Many patients are very well read and insist on using Artemisia treatments. Some have decided to take it in the following manner:

1) Health practitioners from all around the world are recommending 200 mg - 2,000 mg a day of artemisinin depending upon whether it is used for cancer, malaria or chronic Babesia. High doses are divided to keep the blood level intermittently high. Also, it is important to recall that artemisinin induces its own metabolism. **After only 5 days the blood levels fall to one-fifth of the dose found**

on day one.[279] This artemisinin enzyme induction begins just two hours after the very first dose.[280] However, despite this induction in the liver causing artemisinin to be removed very quickly, **the active metabolite, dihydroartemisinin, rises with repeated treatment.**[281]

So in summary, the potent and active metabolite of artemisinin is dihydroartemisinin, and regardless of what happens to artemisinin levels, the potent metabolite climbs. Because of this, I lean toward giving medication breaks so that the dihydroartemisinin level is not constantly high.

2) Some of our patients decide to take oral artemisinin at **25 mg per kilogram per day** divided into two or three doses and **taken two days in a row with one day off**, then restarted. In other words, it is taken for two days, skipped for a day, and then taken for another two days. They may use this dose for months or seasons. This dose is usually between 1250-2500 mg per day depending on their body weight. They also make sure their iron levels are in the top 50% of normal. **Some allopathic physicians are "prescribing" 1800 mg per day of artemisinin.**

3) A malaria web site reports "400 to 800 mg per day can generally be used for at least 6 to 12 months. After that, it can be tapered off slowly." They also report that some believe artemisinin should be taken with food such as cottage cheese or fish oil to enhance absorption.[282]

Since Artemisia products make parasite-killing oxidants or "sparks," it is possible you should not take your antioxidants, such as vitamin C, within 2-1/2 hours of taking an Artemisia product or you might undermine its effect on Babesia. However, how to balance taking free radical making Artemisia products together with protective anti-oxidants in the real world of clinical medicine needs additional research.[283]

4) Oral artesunate is available from HEPAPRO.COM in 400 mg capsules. The **Chinese herbalist, Dr. Zhang, suggests taking 400 mg three times per day and sincerely reports no *serious* side effects.**[284]

Unfortunately, most of the relevant English research studies generally use 500-800 mg per day. Therefore, I personally do not feel that artesunate's safety has been proven at 1200 mg per day taken **daily** for months. I certainly could be wrong, but personally, if I were using this product, I would probably start by using 400 mg three time a day every other day for two weeks. If I did not have complete improvement of my severe fatigue, chills, fevers or sweats, then after fourteen days I would increase it to **two days in a row with a break every third day for up to 6 months.** A few researchers have made the important point that the injury to the hearing centers and brainstem might be so subtle that only sophisticated lab testing would discover it, so I am just trying to be careful.

Oral artesunate doses should be limited to 400 mg at a time, and should not be doubled up in the same day if you forget a dose. Why? We do not have enough studies on dosing variations in humans to know the ideal or the safest single dose. Further, my concern is based on noting that some research seems to show the higher the dose, the higher the risk. It might be that patients taking anti-oxidants or who have a good immune system have little or no risk of side effects. But physicians need to assume the worst.

Therefore, perhaps patients should be offered the option of an audiology exam before starting an Artemisia product, and then offered a repeat audiology exam after two months of treatment. If a patient is too tired to get this testing done twice, then you might consider getting an audiology exam **after taking any Artemisia product for 3-4 weeks** to see if you are developing subtle injury. While this is not the standard of care, I am just trying to be extra careful.

5) World Health Organization (WHO) dosing recommendations are based on the treatment of malaria, not Babesia. But since the two are both parasites that live inside red blood cells, it is useful to read their suggestions.

They believe that it is best to combine any form of Artemisia with a traditional synthetic medication to prevent relapses and to reduce the chance of Artemisia medication resistance in which the Artemisia drug loses its effectiveness over time.[285,286]

- The WHO organization dosing suggestions include: artemisinin at 20 mg per kilogram on the first day, and then 10 mg once a day for 2 days. This would be taken with an added synthetic medicine like Lariam. (Another synthetic medicine, *lumefrantrine*, is going to be aggressively used by the WHO with artemisinin derivatives. This medication is currently not available in the United States).[287,288]

Just as a reminder, the conversion to pounds is:

Kg x 2.2 = pounds.

So a person who weighs 68 kilograms weighs 150 pounds. (150 pounds divided by 2.2 = 68 kilograms).

- Another WHO dosing option is artesunate or artemether dosed at 4 mg per kilogram once a day for three days. Lariam or another synthetic medication with long-lasting effects would need to be added.

If for some reason the second synthetic drug was not going to be added, then the Artemisia product would be used for seven days and not just three days. If artemisinin is used, the WHO suggests 20 mg/kg on day one and 10 mg/kg for six days. Artesunate or artemether would be given at 4 mg/kg on day one, and 2 mg/kg for six days.[289,290]

In future editions, I will most likely revise these dosing guidelines as new information appears. New information should include the best dosing to treat Babesia, and not simply plugging in malaria dosing and assuming it is optimal treatment for Babesia. (Cancer research is currently examining artemisinin products for many types of cancer. Probably, different tumors will require special dosing, frequency, duration and a specific derivative).

In conclusion: I am not offering a cookbook ideal dose for each person for all of Artemisia's medical uses. **So I am referring you to your health care provider to determine your ideal dosing plan. We do not know with certainty how many times a day to safely take Artemisia products.** One study reports that since the blood duration of the active artemisinin ingredient of dihydroartemisinin is fairly short, oral dosing should be **at least twice a day** to maintain an effective intermittent blood level.[291]

If possible, I think three doses causing three blood level peaks might be even better. These three high doses pulsed throughout the day seem to clearly kill malaria and probably Babesia as it enters a vulnerable phase.

Artemisia Sources

The actual dose in a capsule depends on many factors. In Africa and parts of Asia, many capsules have little or none of the active ingredient, but some products exist with good potency and quality. For example, Allergy Research Group tests the potency of every batch they sell.

There currently exists a wide range of types of seeds and locations to grow Artemisia. Artemisia's potency varies from one manufacturer to another based on height, sun exposure, soil, seed variety and time of harvest. Based on these factors, the potency of each batch of artemisinin should be determined by a third party. The purity should also be determined to make sure metals and pesticides are not present.

See Artemisia and Its Derivatives Informed Consent in Appendix F.

Other Medications

Heparin

Heparin is used routinely in medicine to prevent unwanted blood coagulation. It has also been found to limit malaria growth in rhesus monkeys and Babesia in mice. In one study, it was found that B. microti was "significantly inhibited" in the presence of heparin. Treatment with heparin showed complete clearance of Babesia. Heparin **covers the**

surfaces of one stage of Babesia which prevents them from entering red blood cells. My concern with this treatment is that some mice died from the higher doses used. It is not known what is the ideal human dose. Very high dosing could cause excess bleeding or other side effects, but this is a medication with many years of routine and safe use in hospitals. In my three interviews with Babesia experts above, none mentioned using heparin.[292,293]

Quinine

Quinine has a long history of use in the treatment of malaria. Indeed, one pathologist told me she thinks carbonated quinine water (tonic water) may hinder malaria and Babesia. I have not researched this option. Quinine kills Babesia by increasing the pH within Babesia's cells and possibly by dysrupting Babesia DNA.

Quinine Risks

This medication cannot be used in patients with optic neuritis (eye inflammation), ringing ears or a special genetic illness called, "G-6-PD deficiency" (See Appendix B). It should also be used with caution in those with a tendency for white infection cell decreases (granulocytopenia) and patients with cardiac arrhythmias. Do not ignore mild side effects which increase in severity, since very high dosing has a wide range of dangerous side effects, e.g., coma, seizures and death.

Prolonged treatment or overdosing with quinine may cause cinchonism, which is quinine poisoning.

Quinine Side Effects

- Headaches
- Nausea or vomiting
- Blurred vision
- Double vision
- Ringing ears
- Indigestion
- Fever
- Flushing
- Itching
- Low platelets
- Increased liver enzymes or hepatitis

Drug Interactions with Quinine

Quinine affects **five** types of liver enzymes. Therefore, do not take this medication without looking at your current medications and seeing if it interacts with Quinine. It is virtually impossible for a physician to recall all the interactions with this medication. Of course, many of the interactions reported may be trivial.

Some sample interactions are listed below:

- Cimetidine increases quinine blood levels and can cause toxicity.

- Acetazolamide or sodium bicarbonate may increase toxicity by increasing quinine blood levels.

- Quinine may enhance the anti-clotting ability of warfarin and other oral anticoagulants which may cause you to bleed too easily.[294]

- Heart functioning can be disrupted by an increase in beta blockers, tricyclic antidepressants and lidocaine. The heart rhythm medication, digoxin, can increase with quinine and might need to be reduced 50%.

- Aluminum-containing antacids can decrease quinine levels.

- Rifamycins decrease quinine concentrations by increasing hepatic clearance of quinine. This effect can continue for days after the removal of Rifamycins.

- Pain medications such as oxycodone, hydrocodone, codeine and tramadol can decrease when taking quinidine.

Pregnancy and Quinine

Pregnancy category X means it cannot be used during pregnancy.

Quinine Dosing

- 650 mg orally three times per day in adults

- 10-25 mg/kg/day orally in children

Clindamycin

Clindamycin is an antibiotic used to kill many types of infections. It is sometimes combined with quinine to kill maleria and Babesia. Some research reports up to 2000 mg of clindamycin per day is tolerated for 14 days in healthy volunteers, except that such high doses increase gastrointestinal side effects such as indigestion, nausea and diarrhea.

No significant levels of clindamycin are attained in the spinal fluid which circulates all around the brain, so it is probably not directly able to kill malaria or Babesia in the brain.[295,296]

Clindamycin Side Effects

- Upset stomach
- Vomiting
- Gas
- Diarrhea
- Dry skin
- New redness or irritation on your body

- Peeling skin
- New itching or burning of the skin
- Belly pain
- Increased liver function tests

Clindamycin Risks

- Diarrhea with shedding clots or tissue is an emergency
- Skin rashes can be a sign of an emerging dangerous reaction, so call your physician immediately.
- Yellowing of eyes and skin (jaundice) – monitor liver function labs.
- Various infection cell changes – monitor with a CBC test.
- Joint aches which might be a reactive arthritis
- The 75 mg and 150 mg capsules contain FD&C yellow no. 5 (tartrazine); which may cause allergic reactions (including asthma).

Clindamycin Drug Interactions

Clindamycin can increase the function of neuromuscular blocking medications. Therefore, it should be used with caution in patients receiving such agents. Clindamycin and erythromycin may interfere with each other, so these two drugs should not be taken at the same time.

Pregnancy and Clindamycin

Pregnancy category B (See Appendix A). Studies performed in rats and mice using oral doses of clindamycin up to 600 mg/kg/day (3.2 and 1.6 times the highest recommended adult human dose) or subcutaneous doses of clindamycin up to 250 mg/kg/day (1.3 and 0.7 times the highest recommended adult human dose) revealed **no evidence** of teratogenicity.

There are, however, no adequate and well-controlled studies in pregnant women. Because animal reproduction studies are not always predictive of the human response, this drug should be used during pregnancy only if clearly needed.

Nursing Mothers and Clindamycin

Clindamycin has been reported to appear in breast milk in the range of 0.7 to 3.8 mcg/mL.

Pediatric Use of Clindamycin

When clindamycin is administered to the pediatric population (birth to 16 years), appropriate monitoring of organ system functions is desirable.[297,298]

Other Medications

Bactrim or Septra

Bactrim and Septra are the same medication. Some doctors use one name or the other. Both names represent a combo of two medicines: trimethoprim and sulfamethoxazole. Each comes as a regular dose and a double dose. They are also called "co-trimoxazole."

These medications are strong enough to kill routine malaria, even in individuals with compromised immune systems such as those with HIV.[299] However, it appears the younger the child the less effective. For example, children under 3 did not do as well as older youths.[300] If a child is older, such as 5-15 years old, the success rate seems to increase with age to almost a 100% cure of malaria.[301] However, regardless of age, if a youth was malnourished, this treatment did not do well.[302]

Bactrim and Septra Mechanisms

Simply, these medications interfere with folic acid reactions so enzymes do not work correctly, and other aspects of the folic acid system are undermined.

Patient Risk with Bactrim or Septra

People with kidney or liver damage should carefully discuss their dosing with their doctor. Individuals with a unique enzyme deficiency called G-6-PD deficiency should take these medications carefully (See Appendix B). If you have a possible folate deficiency from being elderly, or have poor intestinal absorption, use SAM-e, regularly consume alcohol, birth control pills, antacids, anticonvulsant drugs or metformin, you should ask your doctor for a folic acid and a B12 blood level.

While Bactrim or Septra have been used successfully in vast numbers of people, some have had very severe side effects. Some of these include:

- Fatal full body rashes (so stop this medication if you develop a rash and call your physician).
- Liver damage
- Bone marrow damage
- Seriously high potassium can increase with dosing and might cause heart damage.
- Hypoglycemia is possible in older patients and small children.
- Inflammation of the heart
- Seizures
- Neuron inflammation or damage
- Confusion
- Inflamed neck spine tissue
- Muscle breakdown
- Pancreatitis

Bactrim or Septra Side Effects

- Nausea
- Vomiting

- Reduced appetite
- Rash or skin itching
- Muscle aches
- Kidney disease
- Cough, shortness of breath

Drug Interactions with Bactrim or Septra

Both of the medications in Bactrim or Septra cause a liver enzyme called the "2C8/9" enzyme to be less functional in the body. Therefore any medication, herb or nutrient which also uses this enzyme can have an altered blood level. It impacts other liver enzymes also, but this is the most potent. So why does this matter? Because some drugs are altered when you take Bactrim or Septra.

The following drugs are increased with Bactrim or Septra:

Methotrexate

Procainamide

Amiodarone

Fluoxetine

Glimepiride

Nateglinide

Phenytoin

Pioglitazone

Rosiglitazone

Sertraline

Warfarin

ACE inhibitors, angiotensin rceptor antagonists and potassium sparing diuretics may increase the risk of dangerously high potassium

Cyclosporine

Pyrimethamine over 25 mg/week can cause a dangerous anemia

The following drugs are decreased with Bactrim or Septra:

Carbamazepine
Phenobarbital
Phenytoin
Rifampin
Rifapentine
Secobarbital

The use of the herbs dong quai and St. John's wort can cause interactions and a sun sensitivity rash.

Allergies to "Sulfa"

Bactrim and Septra are considerd "sulfa" medications, so if you have been told you have an allergy to other "sulfa" medications mention this to your physician.

Bactrim and Septra Pregnancy Risk

They carry a pregnancy risk factor of C/D since two medications are involved (See Appendix A). This medication undermines folic acid functioning which is a risk to the fetus. Women attempt to reduce low folic acid damage early in their pregnancy with supplements when they are pregnant or might become pregnant. Usually, expert advice is needed if these medications are being used during a pregnancy.

Bactrim and Septra sound like many other medications, so be extra careful with your pharmacist in confirming you are getting the medication that contains: trimethoprim and sulfamethoxazole or is also called "co-trimoxazole."

Bactrim and Septra Dose Form and Size

Liquid forms: Sulfamethoxazole 200 mg and trimethoprim 40 mg per teaspoon.

Regular size: Sulfamethoxazole 400 mg and trimethoprim 80 mg tablets

Double Strength (DS): Sulfamethoxazole 800 mg and trimethoprim 160 mg tablets

Injection options also exist but are outside the scope of this book

Antifungals

Medications used to treat fungal infections are really misnamed. They also can kill Lyme and other infections that are not fungal. From one study on the use of anti-fungals to treat malaria, we find that some have possible utility with parasites like malaria. Specifically, clotrimazole (Mycelex, Gyne-Lotrimin), econazole (Spectazole), ketoconazole (Nizarol) and miconazole (Monistat). However, this research is very preliminary in terms of their use with red blood cell parasites like malaria and Babesia.[303]

Doxycycline

The long-established antibiotic doxycycline, used to treat acne, has also been shown to be effective against chloroquine-resistant malaria, although it is not licensed for this use. A few studies seem to show it has an ability to control or kill Babesia. Specifically, lab animals given a very dangerous type of Babesia canis were treated with a modest dose, and while the doxycycline did not completely prevent clinical disease, the Babesia symptoms remained moderate and surprisingly a full clinical recovery was obtained within 1 week. When the dose was increased, clinical symptoms ended promptly. The possibility of residual Babesia without symptoms could not be ruled out.[304]

In another study, doxycycline was used in dogs with Babesia canis and Ehrlichia and they recovered without any problems. While doxycycline is a routine treatment for an Ehrlichia infection, it is important to note the dogs recovered with Babesia in their blood when only using doxycycline. So perhaps it also has anti-Babesia effects.[305]

In three other studies Babesia was controlled by doxycycline in combination with traditional malaria medications like quinine in two studies[306,307] and clindamycin[308] in another. In another study, it was found that doxycycline was the malaria medication of choice prescribed by Australian physicians for people visiting multiple drug-resistant malaria infested locations from 1998-2002.[309]

However, out of 19 travelers going to a high malaria area who were treated with doxycycline 53% developed malaria. So a question exists if this has strong utility for malaria and also for Babesia.[310]

Doxycycline and Pregnancy

Doxycyline is generally not recommended during pregnancies, especially in the last 4-5 months, because it may discolor an unborn infant's teeth and undermine the growth of infant bones.

Breast-feeding, Teeth and Bones and Doxycycline

A nursing infant or a child eight years of age or younger may develop discolored teeth or impaired bone growth.

Drug Interactions with Doxycycline

The following medications interact with doxycycline:

- Birth control pills **might** become less effective. The research is not clear. My recommendation is to always use two forms of birth control if you do not want a child. This is especially true with this antibiotic that might alter birth control pill effectiveness.

- Digoxin levels can increase and this increases your risk of heart death.

- Warfarin levels increase with doxycycline causing a bleeding risk.

- Antacids, calcium or iron supplements, or magnesium products may reduce the blood levels of doxycycline.

- Penicillin antibiotics used with doxycycline might decrease the levels of penicillins, e.g., Amoxicillin, Ampicillin, Piperacillin and Ticarcillin.

Doxycycline Dosage

We do not know the ideal dose for treating Babesia. For the prevention of malaria, adults and teenagers take 100 mg starting two days before arriving at a malaria location and then daily while visiting. One would continue this dose after you return for days or weeks.

Children are dosed at 2 mg/kg once a day in the same manner as adults.

Doxycycline Side Effects

- Sun exposure even for brief periods may cause a skin rash, itching, redness or a severe sunburn.

- High brain pressure

- Inflammation of the heart sac

- Mild to dangerous rashes

- Discolored thyroid gland

- Bloating

- Clay colored stools

- Cough

- Dark urine

- Decreased appetite

- Indigestion

- Ulcers in esophagus

- Diarrhea

- Swallowing discomfort

- Dizziness

- Eosinophilia (high eosinophil blood level)

- Fast heartbeat

- Anemia from burst blood vessels

- Fever

- Headache

- Neutrophils low (blood test)

- Low platelets

- Hives

- Itching

- Puffiness or swelling of any part of the front of the face

- Joint or muscle pain

- Swollen lymph glands

- Tightness in chest

- Unusual tiredness or weakness

- Unusual weight loss

- Wheezing

- Yellow eyes or skin[311]

Plaquenil

Hydroxychloroquine or Plaquanil kills malaria and possibly Babesia by increasing cell pH, interfering with the breakdown of hemoglobin and it hinders two infection cells (neutrophils and eosinophils) which are thought to be involved in autoimmune reactions. It also hinders an inflammation process associated with antibodies and material perceived as foreign (antigens).[312,313]

Plaquinil is used for Lupus and Rheumatiod arthritis, but many forget it is a malaria medication. It is still recommended for a wide variety of malaria parasites. However, it is not considered as effective against malaria that is resistent to chloroquine.[314-316]

Hydroxychloroquine is a 200 mg tablet taken by mouth. When a person is exposed to malaria the treatment lasts *a full 8 weeks after exposure*. Very high doses are given for a couple days if you are clearly infected with malaria, and continued at a lower dose after an initial high bolus treatment.

For lupus, one or two tablets are usually taken each day. For rheumatoid arthritis, one to three tablets are usually taken once a day.

Risks with Plaquenil

You must have an eye exam at least every 6 months with this medication, because it can cause possible severe and possibly irreversible eye damage. If you have new and sudden vision changes please get an eye exam in 24 hours and stop this medication. The recommended "safe" daily dose for hydroxy-chloroquine ranges from 1.6 mg per kilograms (3.5 mg per pound)[317] to 6.5 mg per kilogram of body weight to reduce the risk to the eyes. (As a reminder, kilograms = pounds/2.2).[318-320]

If you have taken a medication like chloroquine (Aralen) or primaquine and it has altered your vision in any manner, it may mean you cannot take this medication.

On rare occassions this medication can damage the heart muscle so it does not function. Similarly, it can damage any body muscle. It has also been found to cause any psychiatric disorder, including ones as severe as psychosis.

Let your physician know if you have liver or kidney disease or if you have a G-6-PD genetic deficiency.[321] If you are not sure about the G-6-PD issue, ask for it to be checked—a simple blood test can rule it out and it is hardly rare (See Appendix B). This is the most common genetic abnormality worldwide and is in millions of people.

Plaquenil Side Effects

- Headache
- Dizziness
- Diarrhea
- Stomach pain
- Vomiting
- Skin rash
- Loss of appetite
- Indigestion

Emergency side effects—go to an emergency room and call your physician immediately.

- Ringing in ears
- Muscle weakness
- Bleeding or bruising of the skin
- Bleaching or loss of hair
- Emotional or cognitive changes
- Irregular heartbeat
- Sleepiness
- Seizures
- New trouble reading or seeing

- Sensitivity to light (you must have sunglasses or your eyes hurt)
- Blurred vision
- Seeing light flashes or streaks
- Difficulty hearing
- Hallucinations
- Confusion[322]

Pregnancy and Plaquenil

If you are not using two forms of birth control faithfully you are open to becoming pregnant. Plaquenil is a Class C medication (See appendix A on ratings). If you become pregnant call your family physician and GYN immediately. According to a Canadian family physician journal, we have limited information on this medication's effects on the fetus. Most of the articles on this drug discuss preventing malaria infections. Such prevention requires much lower doses than those used for joint diseases. These lower doses appear in one article to have minimal adverse effects on the fetus.

Several studies on Plaquinil used for rheumatology diseases during pregnancy, failed to show adverse fetal effects, although in most cases, only first-trimester exposure was reported.[323] In another study, of the 215 reported pregnancies with chloroquine and hydroxychloroquine (Plaquinil) exposure, *only seven (3.3%) had congenital abnormalities.*[324]

Primaquine

In animal Babesia studies, this medication did quite well. Specifically, in comparison against other medications for Babesia felis, Primaquine was superior.

Simply, it is the veterinarian's drug of choice for this type of Babesia which removes symptoms, but does not fully kill the infection. Repeated or chronic therapy may be required.[325,326]

While relapses have been reported with all malaria medications, especially if used for a brief time, this one might have a higher incidence of relapses. However, adding it to other malaria medications has been very successful.[327,328] Further, as a preventive malaria medication in which 106 travelers went to a high malaria location, only 5.7% taking primaquine developed malaria over 3 months after their return. To put this in context, 53% of doxycycline recipients developed malaria, and 52% of the mefloquine recipients developed malaria.[329]

Like some other Babesia and malaria medications, primaquine can cause red blood cells to burst in the 400 million people with an enzyme deficiency. This enzyme helps protected blood cells from being damaged by reactivity. This critical enyzme is glucose-6-phosphate dehydrogenase (G-6-PD) enzyme and is most commonly found in people with Mediterranean, Asian, African and Middle Eastern descent. If you are deficient in this enzyme, your red blood cells can burst if you take primaquine. So patients should be tested by a simple blood test at their routine local lab to see if they have this enzyme deficiency before taking this medication.[330] (See Appendix B).

While my father, an Obstetrician and Gynecologist, feels he did not see that much of this deficiency during his long career, I would suggest anyone with Babesia symptoms or taking any Babesia medication, get this test. Why? **It causes symptoms that resemble Babesia** and it is easily diagnosed. Further, most physicians do not realize that common Babesia treatment medications can cause red blood cell breakdown just like some Babesia species creates. These medications below should be avoided if you are G-6-PD deficient:

Antimalarials:

Chloroquine (Aralen)

Hydroxychloroquine (Plaquenil)

Primaquine

Quinine

Chloroquine (Aralen)

Hydroxychloroquine (Plaquenil)

Dapsone

Methylene blue

Dapsone/pyrimethamine (Maloprim)

Pyrimethamine-sulfadoxine (Fansidar)

Tafenoquine (Etaquine) WR23865

Antibiotics:

Sulphonamides

Co-trimoxazole (Bactrim, Septrin)

Dapsone

Chloramphenicol

Nitrofurantoin

Nalidixic acid

Other common medications and exposures can also cause red blood cells to burst with this common enzyme genetic deficiency. Examples would be:

Aspirin

Moth Balls

Fava or broad beans[331]

As you can see below many of the symptoms of this enzyme deficiency resemble Babesia, which manifest when positive patients take medications like Primaquine. In these G-6-PD enzyme deficient people, destroyed red blood cells can be from Babesia or taking medications that cause red blood cell explosions.

- Abnormal paleness or lack of color of the skin

- Jaundice, or yellowing of the skin, eyes, and mouth

- Dark color to urine

- Fever

- Weakness

- Dizziness

- Confusion

- Intolerance to physical activity

- Enlargement of the spleen and liver

- Increased heart rate (tachycardia)

- Heart murmur[332]

Primaquine Dosing

While primaquine was the most effective against Babesia felis, increasing a dose even a small amount is a concern. For example, injected primaquine was the best and the obvious choice compared against other treatments. The recommended dosage is 0.5 mg/per kg of body weight. Repeated treatments are well tolerated but single doses in excess of 1 mg/kg are known to cause mortality in cats. So while 0.5 mg was effective, doubling the dose was dangerous.[333]

Primaquine Drug Interactions

Primaquine inhibits a liver enzyme called 1A2 that may increase blood levels of aminophylline, fluvoxamine, mexiletine, mirtazapine, ropinirole, theophylline, trifluoperazine and others using this enzyme.

Primaquine levels may drop in the presence of amino glutethimide, carbamazepine, nafcillin, nevirapine, phenobarbital, phenytoin, and other 3A4 "inducers."[334]

Grapefruit juice increases Primaquine levels so individuals on this medication should not drink grapefruit juice.[335] For a complete list of medications that interact or might interact log on to: http://medicine.iupui.edu/flockhart/table.htm.

Other Possible Babesia Medications

Biotoxin Binders: Cholestyramine

In a study by Dr. Shoemaker, he hypothesized that Babesia might have biotoxins just like Lyme does—chemicals with the ability to act on the body in a toxic manner after being released from Babesia. He tried out this hypothesis by treating patients who were positive for Lyme disease and Babesia and who failed a "course of antibiotics" for their Lyme.

These patients had previously tried Mepron, Zithromax, and still showed diffuse neurological dysfunction with a special vision test, the visual contrast sensitivity test.

Patients were treated with either Mepron and cholestyramine or placebo and cholestyramine. The biotoxin binder cholestyramine was used in both groups for 16 weeks. (Patients on sugar pills were crossed over and given Mepron after three weeks so that all patients received significant Mepron and cholestyramine.) While some infectious disease physicians do not want to mix the fatty Mepron medication with the cholestyramine fat binder, in this study it was not a problem. Actually, the opposite occurred. The combination of Mepron and cholestyramine had a clear benefit after nine weeks and **the longer they were on this combination the better they felt,** and the better were their neurology scores on their brain neurology test – the visual contrast sensitivity test. At the conclusion of week 12, 21/25 had markedly improved with a clear reduction in symptoms (16 people) or no symptoms (5 people). It is suggested further treatment would continue these improvements.

Dr. Shoemaker's hypothesis is that cholestyramine was binding some type of neurotoxin made not just by Lyme, which clearly has biotoxins, but also by Babesia. I will defer you to his website for additional evidence on this Babesia theory and biotoxin research at www.chronicneurotoxins.com. I am not taking a position currently on whether Babsesia has biotoxins, and defer to Dr. Shoemaker's future research and other veteran Babesia researchers to determine if Babesia has surface biotoxins. In terms of the success of this important study, some physicians feel it is possible the cholestyramine bound Lyme biotoxins while Mepron killed the Babesia.[336]

The *Lancet* published an article that might be related to this biotoxin question. Since Dr. Shoemaker has catalogued biotoxins from a wide range of sources, such as many indoor molds, some algae, Lyme, certain bacteria, some insects, and many other sources, the possibility that Babesia will be exposed to biotoxins from another organism source is common. In this context, this Lancet study is important. Specifically, mice given various amounts of *bacterial biotoxins,* such as are commonly found in flooded and leaking human buildings, required *a very small* amount of Babesia or malaria to kill them—a several hundred-fold reduction.

Why did this combination kill the mice so powerfully? Some feel this bacteria biotoxin load was added to by Babesia and malaria's biotoxins. Others feel these bacteria biotoxins weakened the parasite so that it died by other means than Babesia biotoxins. The main message for use is that a person with Babesia or malaria cannot live in moldy structures or swim in lakes with biotoxin-making algae. **Any biotoxins from any source plus a Babesia infection is deadly.**[337] If you are interested in various biotoxin binding options, see my *Mold Illness and Mold Remediation Made Simple.*

Anti-Oxidants in Babesia Treatment

Babesia and malaria damage your body with significant red blood cell membrane rigidity. As these infection-filled red blood cells try to squeeze through tiny blood vessels, they get stuck and cause clots. The lower the anti-oxidants, the greater the damage and rigidity of infected red cells. Therefore, it is believed by some researchers that providing anti-oxidants, for example, Vitamin E might help keep red blood cells infected with Babesia less rigid.[338]

Of course, better versions of natural Vitamin E are natural forms and not just a synthetic alpha version. Other anti-oxidants are sold alone such as NAC, Vitamin C, alpha lipoic acid. While others are available in quality mixes of many anti-oxidants like NSI's Occupower. (I offer this and other nutrients at *published wholesale* prices off my website, www.HopeAcademic.com). However, I have never seen a mix of anti-oxidants offer enough NAC, so plan on adding at least two NAC capsules per day.

Does Glucosamine Kill Babesia?

One popular nutrient is reported to undermine a common stage in both malaria and Babesia. Specifically, a special part of malaria is the trophozoites, which are also present in Babesia. A common nutritional product used to help prevent arthritis is called glucosamine, and in malaria this inhibits the trophozoite stage. Therefore, some physicians or patients are considering using this non-FDA approved nutrient for Babesia treatment.   Since the FDA does not allow specific health claims even for essential nutrients the body requires, I will make no promises for glucosamine in Babesia treatment. The dosing one would use is unknown.[339]

New Malaria and Babesia Medications

If I am able to do future editions of this book, I will discuss in detail other treatment options. Since I feel it is important to publish this initial edition now, because it is clear much of this clinical material is unavailable, I will only offer some initial data on medications with promise.

Little money is to be made in malaria/Babesia medications, because malaria is most often a poor person's infection and Babesia is routinely missed world-wide. So there is little drive economically to find new treatments. Nevertheless, let me introduce two that might be of use. One new parasitic medication is available now and is called Alinia (nitazox-anide) and the other is called Etaquine (tafenoquine). The latter is in the final research stages in the United States and has been found to *completely kill and cure Babesia microti* in hamsters.

Alinia (nitazoxanide)

Nitazoxanide is marketed in the United States and in Australia. It seems to be a well-tolerated antiparasite medicine with very broad killing ability since it is effective for intestinal pathological protozoa, dangerous intestinal bacteria, and various worms. It does *not* make free radicals or hurt DNA in the human body, so it is probably less likely to cause cancer or hurt a fetus when compared to most other medication options. It also is unique in the way it kills infectious organisms. The probable main mechanism of effectiveness is through interfering with the PFOR system which is essential for non-oxygen energy metabolism—like what occurs in Lyme.[340,341]

While this medication is thought of as a poorly absorbed medication that is limited to killing infections in the intestines, it is clear 1/3 of the active metabolites are excreted in the urine—which means it is obviously entering the body. Therefore, while most of the active metabolites do not get absorbed, 1/3 do get absorbed and have the potential to have systemic effects. Currently, the plasma blood levels of the two active metabolites seem to be on the low side, measured in micrograms, so one question is what blood level is needed to achieve the death of infections such as Babesia, Lyme or others.

In my contact with the maker, they report being told by some physicians that it may help kill both Babesia and Lyme disease. In a recent medical conference, individual physicians mentioned they are beginning to use this medication to treat Babesia and they feel they are having good results. Of course, these are unpublished comments discussing an off label use. I defer this issue to you and your health care practitioner.[342]

Some clinicians think avoiding the anti-oxidant CoQ10 while using this medication is important because it *might* undermine the mechanism of its infection killing.

Alinia becomes tizoxanide or tizoxanide glucuronide. This might be important in the future to ***measure your blood levels*** to see if you are a slow, normal or very fast metabolizer. This is rarely done with important medications or herbs for reasons that elude me. Currently, it appears only the manufacturer can measure these levels.

Food increases the blood levels markedly.

This medication requires a healthy liver, a healthy gallbladder, and healthy kidneys for good excretion. If one of these organs are injured, your blood levels might need to be adjusted.

Alinia Dosing Options

• Alinia Tablets come in 500 mg

• Alinia liquid comes in 100 mg per teaspoon (5 mls)

Alinia: Infant and Adolescent Dosing

The liquid form at 100 mg per teaspoon has been tried on infants as young as 1 year. The 500 mg tablets have been used in adolescents.

Babesia Dosing with Alinia

Some other parasites are being treated in infants with 100 mg teaspoon every 12 hours for three days, and 500 mg tablets every 12 hours for three days for adolescents. The idea all infectious agents will need the same dose seems unreasonable. We have no idea what the correct dose might be to treat Babesia or Lyme disease. Of course this assumes that the anecdotal reports of some success against both are true.

Pregnancy and Alinia

This medication is classified as a Category B (See Appendix A). Very high dose studies on rats and modest dose studies on rabbits have not demonstrated injury to these mammal fetuses or to their fertility. No adequate and well-controlled studies exist in pregnant women. Before taking this medicine use two forms of birth control or you have decided to risk a pregnancy while on this medication. If you become pregnant inform your gynecologist and family doctor within 24 hours.

Breastfeeding and Alinia

It is not known whether this medicine passes into breast milk. We know most medicines pass into breast milk in small amounts. Yet many of them may be used safely while breast-feeding. Do not use this medication while breastfeeding unless you discuss this with your health care professional.

Alinia Side Effects

In about 3-6% of patients these four side effects were found:

- Abdominal pain
- Diarrhea
- Headache
- Nausea

Occasional Side effects:

- Belly pain
- Chills
- Back ache
- Flu feelings
- Dizziness
- Sleepiness
- Insomnia
- Discoloration of the eye
- Ear ache
- Lung discomfort
- Sore throat
- Rapid heart rate

- Fainting
- High blood pressure
- Muscle aches
- Leg cramps
- Fractures
- Tremor
- Tingling
- Allergic reaction
- Fever
- Pain
- Heightened senses, e.g. touch
- Vomiting
- Decreased eating
- Indigestion
- Excess gas
- Constipation
- Dry mouth
- Discolored urine
- Pain during urination
- Abnormal period
- Pain in the sides
- Increased ALT (a liver lab test)
- Yellow coloring/jaundice
- Anemia
- High white infection cells
- Rash
- Itching

Some of these side effects above were found at the frequency of placebo sugar pills.

Alinia Drug Interactions

Tizoxanide, the metabolite of Alinia, is markedly connected to blood proteins at a rate approximating 100%. Therefore, one should be careful about using this medication with other medications which are also tightly bound to blood proteins. Examples of other medications with this protein-binding competition problem, would be the blood thinner warfarin used to prevent strokes and dangerous blood clots.

Drugs which are highly protein-bound and might theoretically be altered when combined with Alinia include cardiac, anti-seizure, anti-mania agents and anti-psychotics. A small sample would include:

phenytoin

phenobarbital

nimodipine

warfarin

clozapine

indomethacin

buspirone

propranolol

valproic acid

meloxicam

Liver Drug Interactions and Alinia

This appears to not be a major problem. In terms of "cytochrome P450" enzyme interactions, none were found in lab studies. Use in patients will need to be monitored.

Etaquine (tafenoquine) WR238605

It is common to confirm Babesia infection with the use of rodents like hamsters. In one hamster study using many Babesia treatment options, the researchers were searching for a full Babesia cure. Some familiar United States or International medications used for Babesia were tried such as mefloquine (Lariam), halofantrine, artesunate and artelenic acid – they did not completely cure Babesia at the doses used. Of great importance, **tafenoquine (Etaquine) treatment produced complete death to Babesia microti pasasites.** Blood drawn from Babesia microti infected hamsters, who had been treated with tafenoquine, did not cause any Babesia infections when injected into new healthy hamsters. This is a stunning finding and appears to offer the hope of a complete cure.[343]

Tafenoquine Basics

Tafenoquine, a much-anticipated drug related to primaquine, is now in phase III clinical trials for use in malaria. It is highly convenient to use, and is very long acting, and does not need to be taken daily. It takes 2 weeks to reduce its blood level 50%.[344,345]

Like primaquine, it can cause severe red blood cell breakdown in individuals with glucose-6-phosphate dehydrogenase deficiency. Thus, it is necessary to screen for this condition before beginning the drug with a simple blood test.[346] (See Appendix B).

The majority of studies have also shown it is **highly effective** in preventing and treating malaria which may apply to its killing ability of various forms of Babesia.[347,348]

According to two articles in the *Journal of Infectious Diseases,* tafenoquine is "safe, well tolerated, and effective in preventing" malaria infection and relapse over a wide range of malaria forms over 6 months of exposure and assumed infection. Further, it acts rapidly and does not show signs of resistance.[349-351]

Further, unlike primaquine, tafenoquine has a special ability to accumulate in the very cells that need it to fight malaria and Babesia—red blood cells.[352]

Tafenoquine Pearls

1) Women have a 1.3 fold higher blood level than men. So dose adjustments may need to be made based on gender.[353]

2) The American military and other militaries have spent tremendous time and money trying to find anti-maleria agents to protect their troops. The Walter Reed Army Institute of Research (WRAIR) developed mefloquine (Lariam) and other anti-malaria agents. Actually in association with SmithKline Beecham, WRAIR developed tafenoquine for preventing and treating malaria in deployed military personnel.[354]

Already, field trials to date indicate that tafenoquine is efficacious and can be taken weekly or perhaps even less frequently.[355]

3) Tafenoquine is so effective that doses as low as a single 600-mg dose may be useful for prevention of malaria. Some suggest a loading dose for malaria prevention of 400 mg daily if one is going to be exposed to malaria. The follow up weekly effective dose can range from 50 mg to 400 mg per week. This relates to Babesia because traditionally we consider malaria dosing when treating Babesia.[356-358]

4) Tafenoquine was developed initially as a primaquine alternative. It appears to have been successful because it kills multiple forms of malaria at much lower doses than primaquine. Specifically, a dose of about 3 mg/kg/day for a single week cured monkeys, and 1 mg/kg/day cured 9 out of 12 monkeys. In contrast, primaquine was only partially curative at 10 mg/kg/day for a week.[359]

5) Blood levels will hopefully become available at routine

labs, because rare patients have blood levels that fall below effective dosing. For example, in one study 104 Thai soldiers took 400 mg of tafenoquine daily for 3 days followed by 100 mg weekly for five months. The mean blood level fell each month in this order: 223, 127, 157, 120, and 88 ng/mL. ***Only 1 soldier developed malaria during the study. At the time of malaria diagnosis, his plasma tafenoquine concentration was a mere 40 ng/mL—a fraction of the other patients.*** Therefore, since it is possible for blood levels to fall quite low, I think when treating Babesia or malaria, that trough blood levels should be monitered if possible.[360]

6) Tafenoquine's relationship with Artemisia herbal derivatives is complex. In one study, a 1:1 combination with tafenoquine-artemisinin combination was far more potent than tafenoquine alone. The effective concentrations went from tafenoquine at 210 nmol/L to 16 mol/L and 1,400 nmol/L to 84. It appears obvious these two treatments are synergistic and a very powerful combination.[361]

7) Zithromax is a routine combination with first line Babesia medications like Mepron. If tafenoquine is combined with Zithromax, it makes for a more potent treatment.[362]

Possible Future Anti-Babesia Plant Treatments

Earlier in this book, we discuss the use of the fern Artemisia to treat Babesia. Yet other plant extracts are being explored which have significant Babesia anti-parasite effects. A small sample which have anti-parasitic effects specifically against Babesia include:

Calophyllum tetrapterum
Garcinia rigida
Lithocarpus specis
Sandoricum emarginatum
Shorea balangeran[363]

Can I Pass Babesia to My Infant in the Womb?

Despite the trouble with diagnosing the many human Babesia species, some cases of infant Babesia are published that report that the infant was infected in the womb. Approximately nine cases of congenital Babesia have been published. The real frequency is unknown and outside the scope of this book. Transmission through blood transfusion is also possible, along with tick bites in infants just days or weeks old. Further, since malaria is passed from mother to infant in the womb, it should not be a surprise that the same thing can happen with malaria's cousin, Babesia.[364-366]

Babesia Fatigue Options

The severity of Babesia fatigue in some patients is staggering. An individual who would be wired and have insomnia on one cup of coffee, struggles to be alert and sleep less than nine hours with a Babesia infection. The following options are what many patients have used with success. These options depend on your ideology of treatment and medicine. If you are going to use supplements, I would strongly suggest you consult a progressive nutritionist, a nutritionally literate physician, a doctor of naturopathy or a chiropractor on the best books that offer the risks and benefits of supplements. While nutrients can be very useful, if someone does not know the risks of too much of a supplement, they do not know supplements.

1) Coffee—this can be effective in some, but it can irritate the intestines, cause emotional irritability, and cause diarrhea with high doses.

2) Nicotine patches, sublingual tablets, nicotine gum, compounded nicotine throat inhalers and nicotine nasal inhalers. If nicotine is used, read a few articles on it and try not to allow your blood pressure to reach above 145 systolic or 90 diastolic. Your pulse should also not be over 90. If you have high blood pressure when not taking nicotine, it might be due to the effect of tick infections on your regulatory system and you might benefit from 50 mg magnesium lozenges under the tongue. They are

very effective at lowering high blood pressure.

3) Cytomel or Free T3 Thyroid – Thyroid drops as we age and this probably contributes partly to fatigue and melancholy feelings in some people. However, supplementation usually does not help Babesia fatigue unless the Free T3 thyroid is actually hypothyroid.

4) Creatine – some debate whether this is a useful supplement. All I can report is some patients feel that this helps them if they use it in the morning and early afternoon. Please read the risks and benefits before using, and start with a low dose initially.

5) CoQ10 – we offer this on my web site, www. HopeAcademic.com at full wholesale prices. I mention that because this natural body substance is expensive. Perhaps try a bottle of 50 mg and take one every hour to test your capacities. If you do not become agitated, consider 100 mg every hour until alert. This is a natural anti-oxidant.

6) NADH – this is like CoQ10 in that both make the gasoline of the body, ATP, but we have not had as much success with this one as with CoQ10.

7) L-Acetyl Carnitine – this supplement is also reported to help with energy. Try a standard dose first thing upon awakening, and then take an additional one every 90 minutes if necessary.

8) Provigil – this is a selective alertness medication which is a selective stimulant considered safe even for very fragile elderly patients. It appears to be safe. The dose I would start with is 50 mg, which does not exist, so I would cut the tablet. If you do not have anxiety in 90 minutes and are still not alert, consider taking 50 mg every 90 minutes up to 400 mg. Some physicians might dose this higher if it shows some possible initial benefit. Another issue is cost since many insurance companies like to play games with you and your physician, and reject this exceptional medication that is respected and supported by many physicians.

9) Stimulants such as Ritalin and Dexadrine – these have some risk of heart attacks, liver damage and strokes, but I have yet to see any such severe effects and the fact is that for some Babesia patients they are the only reason they are not fully disabled. They are the only Band-Aids that allow them to function, be alert, focus and complete any task. All medications have some risk, but these have many studies showing they are typically safe to use.

Nevertheless, get an EKG before starting them and also some basic lab work that includes a liver panel and a CBC. Ritalin is the weaker of the two and the one I would use first. Generally, moving in 2.5 mg units and taking it 2-3 times a day is what is required. If you need to use 80 mg of Ritalin per day, you should try Dexadrine options since they are both cheaper and more potent. Patients need to realize that physicians are happy to not write for these controlled medications since anti-patient DEA agents, media hungry Attorney Generals and the Justice department are highly involved in the practice of medicine. They can be amazingly simplistic and authoritarian on the dosing of stimulants. They actually sometimes use their authority to practice medicine without a degree or license. They might decide what is an "excess dose" for you to get out of bed and function. So if you have an anal relative who thinks it is "wrong" for you to use these, I would suggest you have this relative come and care for you 24/7 and provide for your income. I did not think so.

Uneducated critics with a teaspoon of knowledge, rarely have the willingness to help out, since all their energy is spent criticizing those who do and try to heal. If you are given either of these prescriptions do not lose them and do not fill them at a strange pharmacy, since your insurance company and the DEA will be tracking these scripts, and will not assume you were filling them at a store that had them in stock or was close to your work. Your motives can easily be questioned and anything that is out of the ordinary, will have you being looked at like you are part of some international drug cartel.

Be prepared for relatives, pharmacists and some other physicians to criticize the use of stimulants to help you function. What they do not know could fill the universe. Ask them what their real solution is instead, and generally it will be some overpriced "special" energy formula with plant stimulants or some clique solution.

If your relatives are not supportive of your care, your physician might terminate your care or at least stop prescribing stimulants to help you. Critical relatives, state board lawyers, and politically appointed physicians on these boards, the DEA, Attorney Generals and the Justice Department often feel they are medical experts on your illness. They also act as if they are your personal physicians. These agencies and individuals liberally use their power to limit your medical care. For some of them, they would prefer you die in a car accident from poor focus and attention, than take a stimulant. They now have the power to define the medicine you are allowed to receive.

If you have any depression, **never use stimulants to treat any degree of depression**—they are not meant to treat depression, and you will burn them out, and require higher and higher doses. Soon all you will get is side effects with no benefit. Always treat depression **fully** before any ADD-like symptoms or fatigue.

Probiotics

If you have Babesia or Lyme disease most individuals use some natural or synthetic antibiotic or anti-Babesia medication. If you use traditional antibiotics or herbal variations, you need a probiotic. Antibiotics kill the huge numbers of required good bacteria in your 30 feet of intestines. These good bacteria killed with treatment need to be replaced with good bacteria or probiotics. The most commonly used probiotic is yogurt mixed with corn syrup. These are simply junk. Generally, these yogurt type products have bacteria that simply pass through the intestines. In stool cultures I have done, we have **not** found yogurt bacteria binding the intestinal wall and then proliferating. These two steps are critical for a probiotic to be useful:

1) It must bind the gut wall.

2) The probiotic must reproduce itself at a high level.

In the context of antibiotics and anti-Babesia medications, these are issues to be aware of during your treatment:

1) Consider taking prescription Nystatin tablets 500,000 IU tablets 2-3 per day to prevent intestinal and vaginal candida. This is not a probiotic, but it prevents yeast growth. In contrast to other antifungals this one never leaves the intestinal track. If you develop white candida in the back of your mouth, take two teaspoons of some prescription liquid Nystatin and swish it in the back of your mouth for a minute, gargle it for 30 seconds and then swallow it at least once per day, and discuss your immune system functioning with your physician.

2) In the rare event Nystatin does not cure that throat problem, consider mixing some Metagenics or Natren

probiotic **powder** with water and gargling these good bacteria in the back of your throat. I only have 1/200 patients that need to deal with this issue. If you do not have the powder option handy, consider opening some dry capsules and mixing with warm water and gargling with it.

3) Years ago I had some probiotics with a number of impressive sounding bacteria with colonies in the billions. I had some patients stop them for four days and then we did some stool samples. The results were stunning. Their stool had *none of the good bacteria present*. So obviously the bacteria were:

   a. not present initially

   b. died over time in the warm bottle

   c. they were not adhering to the intestinal wall, so they were simply being pooped out

   d. the bacteria were present but not proliferating or reproducing

Therefore, I only use probiotics with documented strains that have been found to be effective. Most probiotics are junk. Here is what we are currently using:

Theralac—this has 5 high dose stains in an enteric-coated capsule. If you have throat or stomach trouble do not use this one alone because it does not open until past the stomach.

Natren Healthy Trinity—this has a long history of effectiveness and has a small release of bacteria in the stomach. I generally use their Healthy Trinity. This is available at the published wholesale price off my web site, www.HopeAcademic.com.

Natren's Gy-Natren—this is specially designed for use in women prone to vaginal yeast infections. If you are this type of person, use this every night before starting any antibiotic or anti-Babesia medication. (This is available at wholesale at www.personalconsult.com).

Metagenics—We use their Ultra Flora Plus DF Capsules. Some of their products use the sugar FOS, but while this does grow good bacteria, it also grows yeast, so I would not get any Metagenics product with it. This is not enterically coated, so it is possibly useful for the stomach. We use with anyone with stomach complaints.

Florastor—this is a very popular yeast that is recommended for children and adults. It is a top probiotic in the world. (This is available at wholesale at www.personalconsult.com).

Probiotic Game Plan

Generally, if a treatment is causing loose stool or diarrhea, I increase the probiotics. I use 2-3 different brands in everyone. This prevents bad bacteria and diarrhea side effects. If someone has had yeast infections in the past, I start with three different probiotics at a dose of three per meal or 9 capsules per day. If a person likes powders instead, both Natren and metagenics offer powdered forms. Also, if someone is prone to vaginal yeast infections, we start with the Natren's Gy-Natren every night at least 36 hours before any antibiotic is started.

Liver Protection While Taking Strong Babesia Medications

One of the surprises to me about routine MD medical care, is that we learn how to protect the liver from Tylenol overdoses, or excess dry cleaning fluid exposure, but we are never trained in helping the liver handle our strong medications. We are warned to run liver function tests to catch signs of liver injury with strong medications, but never told how to prevent such injury. Indeed, if we made a product that made such a claim, the FDA would attack us for making a specific health claim. One cannot even make a specific health claim for essential nutrients that must be taken into the body for our survival.

Before we talk about liver protection, we should understand what we mean when we talk about detoxification and toxins. Unfortunately these terms are tossed around so much that something simple is made confusing.

For our purposes, lets think of body toxins as merely being of four types:

1) **Gas toxins**—treat with fresh air

2) **Metal toxins**—treat with a chelating agent that binds metals

3) **Petroleum/Plastic/Synthetic chemicals/Medications**—discussed throughout this section.

4) **Biotoxins**—treat with ending your exposure, while adding a special biotoxin binding agent. Also, fix the wide range of inflammation, hormone and protein problems biotoxins cause by giving replacements or agents that reset these three systems.

Gas toxins are simple. If you paint your home or have electronics working, you are being exposed to "off-gasing," and the treatment to pollution is dilution with fresh air.

Metals such as arsenic, cadmium, mercury and nickel can be removed by various chelating agents that have been used for decades.

Our third group is fairly large with tens of thousands of examples. When we found that plastic tubing carrying pure water grew breast cancer as well as estrogen, it was a sign that not all plastic is healthy. When we repeatedly find that the sex organs work abnormally with exposure to herbicides and pesticides, it is obvious that synthetic can sometimes mean unhealthy. Below we will discuss some options to lower your risk of damage with the use of strong synthetic drugs.

Our final group is called "bio-" or "living" toxins. Simply, these are biotoxins from living organisms. Dozens of living things make toxins such as bees, algae in central and northern Florida lakes, fire ants, red tide, stingrays, stinging jellyfish, some types of indoor mold and Lyme bacteria.

Just as a refresher, please note the liver is one of the most important organs in the body. If it is severely injured, you often die. If it is not functioning well, your ability to remove universal toxins is weakened, and it will eventually harm your health in one of dozens of ways. The liver is the site for detoxification of the body, a form of mandatory self-defense. We rarely hear commercials about pills for the liver. It is a weak area in traditional American medicine, so folks tend to think the liver is trivial. Wrong. Its role is massive.

The liver processes carbohydrates, fats and proteins, stores nutrients, controls blood sugar and hormone levels. Bile is made in the liver, which is involved in elimination of various wastes. The liver has a major role in nutrition and is very sensitive to deficits.

Various nutrients are required in order for liver detoxification of common biological and environmental toxins, which we all have in our body, to be carried out efficiently.

If the liver does not have basic nutrients, it will have excess free radicals or "damaging sparks" which cause secondary damage to cells. An adequate supply of key antioxidants and free radical controllers or catchers is therefore essential to prevent tissue damage. Since many Babesia medications cause free radical sparks and also have to be removed from the liver, it is wise to keep it healthy.

Proposed Options to Protect the Liver

The liver has two stages or two "phases" in removing a junk substance.

Surprisingly, often the first modification or the first phase of drug or toxin removal makes it even more dangerous.

That is why the second part of the liver clean-up process is so critical. In this second stage of liver cleaning, called Phase II detoxification, both glutathione and Cal D-Glucarate are absolutely critical. Yet my experience is that **few** people have optimal glutathione or Cal D-Glucarate.

Glutathione

Glutathione was never mentioned to me in medical school. But glutathione is profoundly critical and very important for both parts of liver detoxification.

Since we are all exposed to daily pollutants and many of us have poor dietary sources of glutathione, we are possibly on our way to chronic illness with low glutathione. We also may have possible liver cell damage with strong Babesia medications.

I believe the best way to take glutathione is sublingually, by an inhaler, or IV. Obviously, IV is annoying and expensive. Inhaled or nebulized is likely useful for a former smoker (according to J. Wright, MD), but do not overdo inhaled glutathione or you will feel dizzy. We have been pleased with glutathione tablets or hard jelly lozenges made with natural fruit extracts and placed under the tongue. One physician has reported being concerned that glutathione scars tissue, but we have not heard or seen this problem. Folks who abuse sublingual glutathione get dizzy just like they do with IV glutathione.

One can take pills or capsules of reduced glutathione (ideally with some blue/purple fruit extracts which may make it work better). However, absorption through the intestines into the liver is poor with oral glutathione. However, some feel N-acetylcysteine (NAC) with glutathione helps a small amount of glutathione pass into the liver.

Oral capsules of N-acetylcysteine (NAC) and L-Methionine (an amino acid) increase glutathione in the liver. NAC comes in a number of brand names including Mucomyst, Acetadote and Parvolex. For emergency room overdoses, the dosing starts very high with 150 mg per kg during the first hour given IV. So an average sized man would be given 10,500 mg in the first hour. Nebulized doses are just a little less. So obviously NAC is used in emergency rooms routinely at very high doses to help the liver when a person has overdosed on Tylenol or specific dry cleaning solutions. NAC sold in health food or nutrition stores usually comes in 500 or 600 mg capsules – a fraction of emergency doses.

NAC side effects include occasional fever, chills, drowsiness, nausea, vomiting, breathing spasm, low blood pressure, itching, rash, swelling and dizziness. These side effects are rare in my practice because our average liver protection dose is 1,000 to 1800 mg per day (typically 2-3 capsules/day), not ten times this dose as is used in drug overdoses.

Alpha Lipoic Acid also helps revitalize glutathione, but it also lowers your blood sugar. For some this is a good "side effect" since their blood sugar is already too high. Alpha

Lipoic Acid is also an important anti-oxidant free radical catcher. So it would help decrease Babesia red cell membrane rigidity in the same way NAC decreases this problem.

Low body levels of magnesium cause decreased levels of glutathione. In my magnesium research, in which I took cells taken from under the tongue to measure intracellular levels, I have found virtually everyone's body magnesium is poor, perhaps due to the routine calcium in the American diet that displaces magnesium.

NAC creates glutathione for both phase I and phase II liver detox reactions, so it is very important. Glutathione placed directly into the bloodstream is also an exceptional liver protectant nutrient. We use sublingual or nebulized (mist) glutathione to increase blood levels. The sublingual forms come in gel-like sublingual squares with tangerine or blueberry natural fruit oil at Lionville natural pharmacy at 877-363-7374 (Fax number is 610-363-5707). I also use College pharmacy in Colorado to make hard sublingual orange tablets. Their phone numbers are 800-888-9358 or 719-262-0022. Their fax numbers are 800-556-5893 or 719-262-0035. Some physicians use high dose IV Glutathione and this has been reported to be helpful.

Some physicians have reported that only their pharmacy and only their approach can give you good blood levels of glutathione. This is nonsense and arrogant. Many physicians have found that sublingual, nebulized and transdermal cream glutathione has clear side effects which match high doses of IV glutathione, so it is obviously entering the body as expected according to advanced compounding pharmacy techniques. For example, IV glutathione can make you a little dizzy. We have found that our 250 mg sublingual troches can also make someone dizzy every time they take three at a time. Further, we have found certain bad heavy metals that are heavily bound to glutathione are removed in direct proportion to the number of sublingual glutathione troches taken the day of the testing. IV is not the only option. But since many talented physicians are not trained in advanced compounding pharmacy options, these options that deliver medication or nutrients through the skin, the base of the tongue or lungs do not seem credible to them. This is due to a lack of training and experience.

Calcium D-Glucarate

The second part of liver detoxification is called "phase II" detoxification. It is also considered the special glucuronidation detoxification phase. For phase II detoxification it is important to understand that this detox process can be ruined by bad bacteria excretions. Meaning the excretions of some bacteria undermine phase II detoxification. Then this causes the toxins being sent to the phase II liver machinery to simply recycle all over the body instead of being removed.

Calcium D-Glucarate keeps the glucuronidation detox system working well and removing junk. It fights the effects of the bad bacteria excretions that ruin the system like a "metal rod" in a machine ruins its gears. Calcium D-Glucarate pulls out the rod and lets the liver remove junk. So Calcium D-Glucarate increases toxin removal.

Calcium D-Glucarate is not synthetic since it is in some vegetables and fruits.

The Disaster of Fast Part I and Slow Part II Detox

If you have a nutritional, environmental or genetic weakness that spikes Phase I detoxification, you can start building up toxins that are made more dangerous by the liver's Phase I system. If you add to this a weak and impotent Phase II, you will start damaging the body.

For example, imagine that sulfur and charcoal were medicines entering the Phase I system. They could become dangerous gunpowder on their way to Phase II.

We commonly manipulate these two phases in a good way in American medicine. Here is a summary and sample of foods and drugs can alter liver phases.

Zinc **promotes** Phase I reactions, but not Phase II reactions. Grapefruit juice is given to transplant patients to **limit** Phase I detoxification. Why block Phase I and allow medications to stay unmetabolized? Because cyclosporin, the tissue rejection prevention drug, can stay in the body longer. (Additional important liver detoxification information is available in Appendix G.)

General Nutrition for Liver Function

For the liver to remove toxins you need a wide range of nutrition. Basically, when you are building a house it is helpful to have as many tradesman hands as possible – carpenters, plumbers, framers etc. Ideally, you give the liver and the body wide ranging nutrients, instead of thinking you will build your home merely with an expert landscaper. In the same way, the liver does best with a wide range of minerals, vitamins, amino acids and other nutrients. Any "full" daily supplement should have most of the items listed in Appendix G which offers additional specifics on liver health.

The Simple Bottom Line on Detoxification

If you are like most people you are very tired of taking pills. So if you were going to apply all the material in this book on liver detoxification, you might do the following:

1) Take 250 mg of Glutathione per day under your tongue in a special penetrating sublingual base or 1000 to 1800 mg of NAC per day

2) Take standardized Milk Thistle

3) Ingest one Cal-D-Glucarate per day to keep Phase II liver detoxification working well.

4) Swallow 3-4 capsules or tablets of a good supplement. I personally use wholesale NSI options such as Synergy women's formula or NSI Occupower. You can get them off my site at www.personalconsult.com at wholesale. Please compare the dosing, name brands and cost on my web site with other discount or nutrient store prices.

Ongoing Care if Significant Babesia Illness

Some patients develop low oxygenation and shortness of breath before or after starting treatment. Breathing trouble can be caused by fluid in the lungs from some Babesia species.

Individuals with no spleen are at much higher risk of severe Babesia complications and need extra care. They cannot remove infected red blood cells, so blood oxygen is reduced. An individual with no spleen is at risk for kidney failure, seizures, the shut down of multiple organs, and a coma.

Some times the Babesia infection is so bad that deformed and damaged red blood cells cause fluid in the lungs and death.

Some believe that Babesia has chemical toxins on its outer

membrane surface that may be poorly removed in some patients. These biotoxins may contribute to breathing trouble as Babesia dies off, and releases a biotoxin which hurts your health, e.g., by causing lung fluid, tiny lung clots, and clots all over the body. I do not know whether Babesia has biotoxins. I refer you to www.chronicneurotoxins.com to let you explore this on your own.

Certain cell surface protein patterns or HLA genetic patterns (e.g., 15-6-51, 16-5-51, 1-5) are found in individuals who do not remove Lyme biotoxins easily. This was discovered by Dr. Ritchie Shoemaker and published in *Mold Warriors* and replicated by me. Aggressive antibiotic treatment makes some patients with these gene patterns sicker, if their Lyme biotoxins are not promptly bound up, and many hormones and inflammation chemicals become abnormal if Lyme die-off biotoxins circulate in the body, e.g., MSH, VIP, VEGF, MMP-P, MMP-9, 3Ca and TNF-a.

If you have any of these sample HLA patterns listed above, you will need aggressive cholestyramine. This can be started at 1/4 of a teaspoon twice a day. And as your stomach, esophagus, intestines and body are able to tolerate it, you can increase to 3-4 packets per day in divided doses throughout the day. If you feel nausea in the first 30 minutes after taking, consider stomach agents such as high dose acid blockers or Carafate (sucralfate) which soothe the stomach as you get used to the cholestyramine on your raw stomach. If you feel poorly after a couple hours, it might be due to the removal of bound biotoxins being removed, and then replaced in your bile from other body tissues. As they begin to replace what you bound, you might feel poorly. Reduce the dose to the lowest tolerable level.

If you wonder if you are overly sensitive to Lyme biotoxins or mold biotoxins and if you remove them very poorly, buy *Mold Warriors* by Shoemaker, Schaller and Schmidt. If you are too ill to read easily, and you have seen or smelled mold, or are unsure if you have hidden mold, purchase *Mold Illness Made Simple* from www.HopeAcademic.com as an E-book or from Amazon.com. This book discusses your unique HLA pattern which determines how you handle biotoxins. The test order code to see if you have a raw stomach or other biotoxin symptom is: HLA DRB1, 3-5, BDQ Disease Evaluation LabCorp code 012542. Other labs are able to do this testing but only give you 2 of the 5 parts of the LabCorp results.

A Sample Patient Experience

Amy tested positive at two tick specialty labs. One found positive antibodies for Babesia microti and the other lab found visible Babesia in her red blood cells with special staining. She also had symptoms. She told her family doctor that she was struggling with fatigue, muscle pain, burning sensations, memory and concentration problems. She was also sleeping twelve hours a day. She was told she was "fine and should go to work!"

Another physician who had spent considerable time studying tick-borne infections diagnosed her Lyme and Babesia based on her symptoms and lab results. The physician thought her night sweats, fevers and severe fatigue might be from the Babesia.

Amy was treated for Lyme, and she also had two medications added to treat the Babesia. She took Mepron at 750 mg per teaspoon twice a day with Zithromax 250 mg twice a day and an Artesunate 400 mg capsule three times a day for four months.

Her Babesia symptoms cleared after four months, and her follow up Babesia microti testing was negative.

Prognosis Based on Species

Since most infected American Babesia patients have yet to be diagnosed, it is unknown how they are functioning. Medical problems caused by Lyme and Babesia are routinely blamed on other causes and other medical diagnoses. I think many patients with Fibromyalgia and Chronic Fatigue Syndrome have tick-borne infections like Babesia.

It appears your outcome depends partly on which Babesia strain is present. Generally, the divergens type of Babesia, which is more common in Europe than the United States, has a worse prognosis. Some of the new forms discussed earlier, like Babesia duncani, has a worse prognosis than Babesia microti. Many feel that the United States microti form can be fully treated if it is treated seriously. However, different physicians have very different opinions on what is "full treatment." Some feel complete treatment if achieved in 1-4 weeks. Others feel that since Babesia lives inside red blood cells, and these cells live 4 months, that any treatment should be at least four months. Discuss this with your physician or other health care provider.

The many forms of Babesia listed below are rarely tested for and blood smears are usually poorly done which might catch them. Further, it is unclear if all of them should be treated the same way. Some clinicians feel if microti is causing no symptoms, one might not treat it. I do not like the idea of a red blood cell infection calmly floating in my body – I would treat. Other species are more dangerous, and most physicians would treat. Certainly, they would be treated with malaria medications and other treatments used for Babesia microti. Experts are increasingly reporting they are finding new types of Babesia that do not fit short symptom lists or current testing options. Yet we will need more experience and research to know what treatments are best for each species. Since they are not producing the same symptoms, I would not assume they will all require the same clone treatment plan.

WA1-3

CA1-4

CA5, 6

B. duncani—includes both WA1-3, and CA5,6

MO1

B. odocoilei

EU1

EU?

B. canis

B. bovis

B. microti

B. divergens

B. equi

B. "unidentified"

Reducing Your Risk of Tick Bites

Since Babesia is carried by different ticks, and the most common tick to infect humans is the very tiny deer tick or Ioxodes tick, prevention might be the best medicine. Specifically, preventing a tick bite.

Basic Deterrence and Prevention of Tick Bites

- Avoid endemic areas between the months of early spring until winter.

- Cover skin with appropriate clothing, including tucking long pants inside socks. Wear light-colored clothing so "dirt specks" or deer ticks will be visible.

- Examine skin and pets every day as soon as you return from outside.

- While we appreciate a desire to live in a pesticide-free world, Babesia and Lyme are far more dangerous than pesticides. Therefore, wear a tick repellent such as DEET, especially on skin such as feet, ankles and legs. DEET should never be excessively sprayed at levels in excess of the printed directions.

  Other options exist and are being explored which are more "natural." Currently, these options are outside the scope of this book but are being researched.

- Clothing can be treated with Permethrin (known by such brand names as Permanone or Duranon). This should **never** be applied directly to the skin, but only your clothing. When you apply it to your clothing it can take up to four hours to dry, so try not to apply it at the last minute. This product typically kills ticks on your clothing in under a minute.

Additional Anti-Tick Suggestions and Information

- Deer ticks love shady and moist ground litter, so collect grass clippings and do not create a thin mulch layer in your lawn.

- Ticks climb to various heights based on the tick species and the time of year. They can cling to very low grass, tall grass, brush, shrubs and log piles. They live in lawns and gardens, and love the edges of woodlands.

• Deer ticks do not jump or fly. They never drop from a high perch as you walk under them.

• Avoid contact with soil, leaf litter and vegetation as much as possible.

• Wear enclosed shoes

• Tuck in pants and socks to create a cloth barrier between you and any tick.

• Keep long hair pulled back

• When gardening or otherwise handling soil and vegetation, wear light-colored gloves, checking them frequently for ticks.

• Ticks are commonly in shallow grass, so **avoid sitting directly on the ground or on open stone walls** (which attract small mammals that carry deer ticks.)

• Never "plow through" brush and trees as if you are clearing a path through the jungle. Instead, walk **on cleared, well-worn trails** whenever possible. Walk in the center of paths to avoid contact with infected grass or brush.

• During and after any trip outside spot-check yourself and others frequently for ticks on clothes. If you see one tick, assume there are others.

• After returning to the indoors remove clothes exposed from tick-infested areas and, if possible, wash and dry them to eliminate any unseen ticks.

• Ideally, shower and shampoo soon after a possible exposure.

• Be extra careful to check yourself, your children and any outdoor pets from head to toe for ticks each night before going to bed (nymph deer ticks are the size of a period and adult deer ticks are the size of sesame seeds).

• Any contact with vegetation, including simply playing in a yard, can result in exposure to ticks, so if the temperature exceeds 40° degrees, assume deer ticks are out on grasses, bushes and low-lying trees.

• Outdoor dogs and cats can carry ticks into your home. Your veterinarian can offer suggestions on the use of various products to kill ticks on your animals and to keep their bedding tick-free.

• Sleeping with your pet is generally not recommended, even if your pet is only outside to go to the bathroom. Nymphs easily attach to dogs in one inch of grass.

Tick Identification

I used to be quite cynical about any patient's ability to identify ticks, since deer ticks are so hard to see. And yet some people are able to identify them, especially if they are in "the great outdoors" and skim a patch of them.

My patients have been particularly good at identifying the lone star tick that hunts and pursues people, and which is much larger than a deer tick. See the tick identification images on page 36.

Making a Home Unfriendly to a Tick

70% of tick bites occur on your own property. Here are ways to reduce the number of ticks around your home:

- Keep your lawn mowed

- Remove grass clippings since ticks love a moist dying grass layer.

- Remove any wild looking lawn edges by cutting very low down to the soil or removing these grasses or brush.

- Completely clear brush, leaf litter and tall grass around houses, and any other place near your home.

- Stack woodpiles neatly in a dry location and preferably off the ground. Ask a local exterminator about options to prevent mice from living in these woodpiles, since these mice may carry ticks which can cause infection a significant distance from their nest.

- Keep gardens empty of grass, leaf litter and dead perennials. Burning your leaves and dead grass can be an effective way to control ticks if the temperature is high. Try to avoid

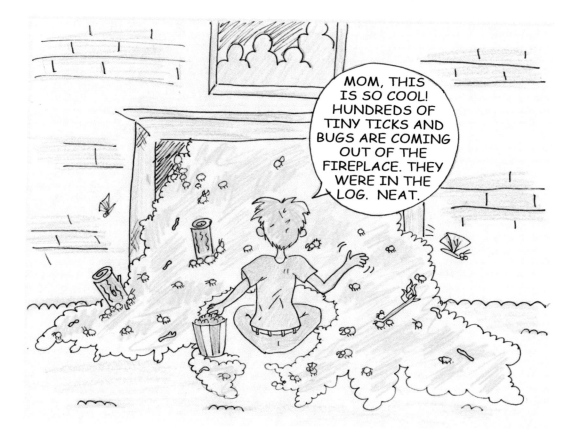

We often feel that if there's any time we are safe from deer ticks its when it is under 40° degrees and snowy. Amazingly there have been clear cases of individuals infected from ticks exiting warm firewood.

creating a 500-acre fire disaster.

- If you are committed to having a bird feeder, remove and clean loose seeds to prevent attracting rodents. Consider asking your local exterminator what might be the best option to spray on these residual seeds deep in the grass which will repel small mammals like mice.

- Consult with a licensed professional exterminator to consider spot spraying on the **edges of your property** to kill ticks in the early spring. Ask about the duration of effectiveness of the pesticide—you might need to do it twice. Make sure the pesticide used is able to kill deer ticks and not some other tick that has less risk of carrying Lyme and Babesia such as the brown tick. Some suggest using pesticides of the pyrethroid class because they are related to the toxins found in some chrysanthemum flowers.

Trained pest experts are trained to use:

- **Damminix** from EcoHealth which are cotton-filled tubes impregnated with permethrin which is spaced every 10 yards or less. The cotton is used to make mice nests and kill the deer ticks they carry.

- **Maxforce Tick Management** by Bayer Environmental has small plastic chambers with the insecticide fipronil which coats the mice and kills up to 96% of the deer ticks in two years.

- **The "four post" deer treatment** in which deer bend down to eat corn, and then rollers apply permethrin. This is spread all over their bodies by grooming. So far it has been found to kill 90-95% of disease-bearing ticks over three years. It requires approximately biweekly corn refilling and insecticide reapplication.[367] This approach typically requires the participation of your entire neighborhood to cover the costs and to have enough feeder stations.

- If you are using DEET and pesticides you might consider looking over the liver protection section earlier in this book. My opinion is that activated pharmaceutical charcoal capsules (or tablets) taken every two weeks on an empty stomach *might* help the body remove absorbed pesticides. Further, taking NAC in capsule or shake form may increase the removal of pesticides you have absorbed.

• Deer fences come in various forms and are outside the scope of this book. They are available in solid 8-foot high options to heavy grade plastic netting to basic and movable electric fences. Confirm your zoning limitations before you erect an 8 ft fortress with a moat. Deer fences appear to be effective *if other small and medium-sized animals are also addressed in addition to the deer.* If the deer are excluded from a yard, but mice, raccoons and skunks have full reign, the deer tick levels will not fall as hoped.

• Some government agencies suggest creating a 3-foot wide, 3-5 inch deep barrier of gravel, woodchips or mulch between your lawn and any wooded area.

• Any play areas or bird feeder areas would also have the same gravel foundation under them and the three-foot barrier around the edge.

• Prune back shade trees very aggressively since the sun will dry up ticks and can kill them.

• Mice that carry deer ticks love stone walls, so make them unattractive by removing loose litter and seal any cracks.

• Natural tick control agents are being aggressively explored by many companies, and I am also researching natural and safe tick control agents such as tick parasites and special fungi and molds. Two options would be parasitic insects that would feed on the tick during some phase of development, and molds or fungi that would kill deer ticks or block some part of the infection cycle.

• Other natural options include everything from various types of tick-eating hens, to mice-eating snakes to the highly aggressive removal and hunting of deer and other possible deer tick carriers.

• Some landscapers believe certain trees, shrubs, vines, bulbs and plants repel deer and these would include: *adromeda, spruce, boxwood, butterfly bush, cottoneaster, leucothoes, spirea, weigela.* For a full listing, go to <u>www.wwhd.org</u>.[368] The American Lyme Disease Foundation home page <u>www.ldf.com</u> also has information.

Appendix A
Pregnancy Classes

Some of the medications mentioned in this book have referred you to various pregnancy "classes" or categories. These each have degrees of pregnancy risk to a developing baby or a level of risk for a birth defect from taking a medication. The FDA reports drug risks in various groupings that run from "Class A" (safest) to "X" (a clear danger – don't use!).

Here is an explanation of these various ratings.

Class A: Reasonably conducted well-controlled studies in pregnant women have *not* shown an increased risk of fetal abnormalities. This is the safest class but an exceptionally rare designation, because we do not test drugs on fetuses.

Class B: This class has two types of meanings.

a. Animal studies have *not* demonstrated a fetal risk. But we do not yet have good human studies in pregnant women.

b. Animal-reproduction studies have shown birth defects, but we do have human studies and the animal defect is *not* seen in the human studies.

Class C: No research studies exist on the effect of this drug in humans. Animal studies have not been done or if animal studies are done, they show some injury to the fetal animal. Some situations might exist in which the risk is outweighed by the need for the medication. This risk versus benefit needs to be discussed and reflected on clearly, because a bad outcome is possible with using the medication or not using it.

Class D: Human data shows risk to the fetus. Nevertheless, there might be situations in which the risk is outweighed by the need of the medication. This risk versus benefit needs to be discussed and reflected on clearly, because a bad outcome is possible with using the medication or not using it.

Class X: Animal or human data shows clear danger to the fetus.[1-4]

Appendix A End Notes

1. From fda.gov: Pregnancy Categories. Available from: http://www.fda.gov/cder/present/dia1-2001/dkennedy/tsld007.htm.

2. From fda.gov: Pregnancy Categories. Available from: http://www.fda.gov/ohrms/dockets/ac/00/slides/3601s2a/sld014.htm

3. Gerard M. DiLeo, M.D. From gynob.com. FDA Drug Risk Classification in Pregnancy. Available from: http://www.gynob.com/fda.htm.

4. From fda.gov: Current Categories for Drug Use in Pregnancy. Available from: http://www.fda.gov/fdac/features/2001/301_preg.html#categories.

APPENDIX B

Babesia and G-6-PD Problems: They Can Look the Same

As many as hundreds of millions of people worldwide have some degree of G-6-PD enzyme deficiency. Why does this matter? Simply, it can cause red blood cells to rupture in a way similar to most species of Babesia. Further, if a person has this enzyme deficiency, medications as simple as an aspirin, and food as basic as a certain bean type, could cause red blood cells to rupture. This deficiency comes in many forms. Therefore, some have no obvious symptoms and some have marked symptoms. So depending on your genetics, it could be that only a very few red blood cells will rupture, or many will rupture. This is one reason this should be checked in anyone with possible Babesia—an infection that ruptures red blood cells and is treated with some medications that may rupture if someone has a type of G-6-PD deficiency.

The test is:

Glucose 6-Phosphate Dehydrogenase (G-6-PD), Quantitative, Blood and Red Blood Cell Count (RBC)

The LabCorp order number is 001917 and requires two tubes of whole blood.

APPENDIX C

Lyme Persistence:
A Sign of Babesia Persistence?

Some sincere infection physicians feel that all Lyme is killed completely with 21-30 days of antibiotics. On my web site, www.hopeacademic.com, we list large numbers of studies showing this is not the case.

In the same way, I am seeing two standards of care for the treatment of Babesia. Some feel it is killed in days, and others think in terms of months. In Appendix D by Dr. Metzger, is a sample of the reasons some physicians treat Lyme until a clear cure has been achieved. Some of the reasoning is similar to the reasons some treat Babesia longer.

❧

APPENDIX D

Late Stage Lyme Disease:
Arguments for an Individualized Approach

Deborah A. Metzger, PhD, MD

The purpose of this review is to provide arguments in favor of a more liberal approach to the treatment of late stage Lyme disease, specifically the use of intravenous antibiotics for extended periods of time.

Lyme disease is a chronic, persisting, multi-systemic infection, which is caused by *Borrelia burgdorferi* spirochetes that are transmitted by common deer ticks (Ixodes). Like syphilis, which is another spirochetal infection, Lyme disease may affect several organ systems and proceed through several stages. It may also persist if it is not properly diagnosed and treated in the earliest stage. During the first stage, a pathognomonic bull's eye rash may develop that establishes the diagnosis. It is often accompanied by a flu-like illness. Unfortunately, in 20-50% of those infected with Borrelia, no rash develops, develops in an uncharacteristic form, or is not noticed[1,2]. Without appropriate antibiotic treatment, the disease becomes disseminated resulting in episodic or persistent neurologic, musculoskeletal, or cardiac symptoms. Several lines of evidence suggest that Lyme disease is very much underreported[3] and that perhaps as many as 90% of those affected are not diagnosed.

Ticks that carry the Lyme bacteria also carry co-infections such as Ehrlichia, Babesia, and Bartonella. Approximately 2/3 of patients with Lyme disease have at least one of these co-infections[4] but patients are not routinely tested for them. Patients who have Lyme disease together with a co-infection may remain mysteriously ill and unresponsive to standard treatment. Thus, Lyme is a complex illness potentially consisting of multiple tick-derived co-infections.

Most physicians agree that when treated very early in the course of the disease that most Lyme patients will get well. Also generally agreed is that Lyme disease patients who have gone undiagnosed and now suffer late stage disease may continue to experience debilitating symptoms following a month-long course of antibiotics. All agree that these symptoms-arthritic, neurologic, and multisystemic-can last for months or years. The most controversial aspect of the treatment of late stage Lyme disease is the optimal antibiotic regimen.

For the vast majority of bacterial infections, a defined course of antibiotics either eliminates the bacteria or decreases the number of bacteria so that the immune system can eradicate the survivors. Lyme disease is not a typical bacteria in that it shares some of the characteristics of more challenging bacterial infections such as mycobacteria and syphilis: it is difficult to routinely culture, has a slow growth rate, can remain dormant for lengthy periods[5], can invade intracellular sites[6,7,8,9], and may sequester in areas where antibiotic penetration is problematic such as the CNS, joint cartilage, and anterior chamber of the eye[10]. To make matters worse, there are no tests that reliably determine when Borrelia has been effectively eradicated. As clinicians, we are left to use our best medical judgment in individualizing care for our patients.

Oral antibiotics are preferred because of the ease of administration and low cost. Intravenous antibiotics are used for infections that are resistant to orally administered antibiotics, when inadequate blood levels are achieved by the oral route, or when penetration into privileged sites (i.e., the CNS) or poorly vascularized tissue (i.e., cartilage) is needed.

Review of the medical literature to determine an evidenced based approach for the treatment of late Lyme disease reveals a paucity of data. The studies that are often quoted as supporting a particular evidenced-based approach to late Lyme disease are summarized in Section 1.

There are several themes that run through these diverse studies:

1. Antibiotics are accepted as mandatory in active Lyme disease treatment. However, the ideal antibiotics, their dosage, route of administration and duration of therapy have not been established.

2. Many patients remain well after a single course of oral, IM or IV antibiotics. However, many other patients with Lyme disease, initially improve while on antibiotics but relapse when antibiotic treatment is discontinued. There is often relief of symptoms when antibiotics are reinitiated, implying persistence of the bacterial infection.

3. Many of the antibiotics used in the studies do not penetrate the CNS, such as doxycycline[11]. Thus, persistence of neuroborreliosis would be expected.

4. The most effective treatments for late Lyme disease include at least 2 weeks of intravenous ceftriaxone or cefataxime. Retreatment protocols, for relapses and treatment failures, include significantly longer treatment courses, i.e., greater than 4 weeks.

5. None of the studies included evaluation and treatment for the co-infections such as Rocky Mountain spotted fever, Babesia, babesiosis, or ehrlichia that are present in as many as 2/3 of patients. This may explain the poor response to treatment in some of the studies using 30 days of IV antibiotics.

6. Persistence[12] of symptoms or relapse is quite common[13,14] implicating that duration of treatment and/or the type of antibiotic used is inadequate. Relapse and failure to respond to intensive antibiotic treatment has been attributed solely

to an autoimmune reaction related to the presence of Borrelia[15]. However, there are studies documenting the persistence of *Borrelia burgdorferi* in antibiotic-treated patients[16] and following up to 12 months of intravenous antibiotic therapy[17,18,19]. Section 2 summarizes the studies that demonstrate persistence of *Borrelia burgdorferi* after antibiotic treatment.

7. Most of the studies involved highly selected patient populations. Lyme patients present with a broad spectrum of symptoms and response to antibiotics. Thus, the relevance of the conclusions of these studies to most patients with late Lyme disease is problematic.

8. Many antibiotic regimens do not take into account that many antibiotics only kill actively dividing organisms. The fact that some cultures of *Borrelia burgdorferi* have taken up to 10 months to grow suggests that most treatment guidelines recommend a too short period of antibiotic treatment.[20]

9. Given the range of symptoms related to Lyme disease and the widely divergent response to antibiotic therapy, treatment needs to be individualized. This means that some patients may require much longer treatment with oral and/or intravenous antibiotics.

10. There is not sufficient evidence from the studies published to date to develop treatment guidelines.

In spite of the paucity of data, two groups of physicians that treat Lyme disease independently developed peer-reviewed 'evidence-based' treatment guidelines using the same literature (Section 1) to formulate their treatment guidelines. The Infectious Disease Society of America (IDSA) advocate a maximum of 30 days of oral or intravenous antibiotics and assume that the remaining symptoms reflect a self-perpetuating autoimmune response[21]. The International Lyme and Associated Diseases Society (ILADS), which is composed of physicians from a variety of specialties who primarily treat Lyme disease, assume that the persistent symptoms reflect ongoing infection and gauge the duration of treatment by the patient's individual clinical response. These physicians believe that there is insufficient evidence at this point to adopt standardized treatment protocols[22].

While each viewpoint has a strong underlying hypothesis, the scientific evidence supporting either viewpoint is equivocal. Outcomes research is limited and conflicting. The NIAID has only funded three double-blind, placebo-controlled treatment outcome studies for long-term treatment of persistent Lyme disease. The findings of two studies (Klempner and Krupp-Section 1) are contradictory, with one indicating that continued treatment is beneficial for treating fatigue and the other indicating that it is not. The third NIAID-funded study

(Fallon-Section 1) has recently been completed and preliminary results support continued antibiotic treatment for patients with persistent Lyme disease. The findings of nine non-controlled studies (Section 1) support continued treatment. The existence of limited or conflicting controlled studies is not uncommon in the practice of medicine.

When a variety of viable treatment options exist, therapy is decided by weighing the individual's risks and benefits. Use of antibiotics can be associated with side effects, allergic reactions, development of drug resistance and cost. The benefits of antibiotics are the relief from a severe multisystemic bacterial infection that is difficult to eradicate with short-term antibiotic treatment. Witholding adequate antibiotic treatment for late-stage Lyme disease (when it is known that Borrelia persist in many treated patients-see Section 2) is analogous to the Tuskegee experiment performed by the Public Health Service[23], which has been widely criticized for the failure to adequately treat African American men with late-stage syphilis, another spirochete disease.

Insurance companies have adopted guidelines reflecting short-term treatment approaches, which are governed by cost-containment considerations. However, the legal standard of care for treating a condition is determined by the consensus of physicians who actually treat patients, not by treatment guidelines[24]. One survey found that 57% of responding physicians treat persistent Lyme disease for three months or more[25].

Fallon notes that for over 3400 patients screened for the Columbia University study of persistent Lyme disease, the mean duration of IV treatment was 2.3 months and the mean duration of oral antibiotic therapy was 7.5 months[26]. In another survey, "50% of the responders considered using antibiotics for a time greater than one year in a symptomatic seropositive Lyme disease patient. Almost that same number would extend therapy to 18 months if needed."[27]

When more than one standard of care exists, the critical question becomes who decides the appropriate course of treatment for the patient. Under the medical ethical principle of autonomy, the treatment decision belongs to the patient. Hence, the American Medical Association requires that the physician disclose and discuss with the patient not only the risks and benefits of the proposed treatment, but also the risks and benefits of available alternatives[28]. Treatment choices involve trade-offs between the risks and benefits of treatment options that only patients, who know the kinds of risks they are willing to run and the types of quality of life outcomes that matter to them, are uniquely suited to make.

Insurance companies have placed the full weight of their economic clout behind the less expensive short-term treatment protocols. More expensive longer-term treatment options are discredited as "experimental" or "not evidence-based." The point, of course, is that the science underlying both the short-term and the longer-term treatment options is equally uncertain. It is estimated that only 20% of medicine practiced today is rooted in double-blind studies.[29] The bulk of medicine today is practiced in the grey zone. Evidence-based medicine requires only that medicine be practiced in accordance with the evidence that currently exists, not that treatment be withheld pending research. As for the cost considerations, health care costs generally are lower when the patient's preference is supported[30].

In an ideal world, decisions would be based on strong scientific evidence, consensus opinion, and the views of the treating physician. However, seldom are all three available. A recent symposium by the National Institute of Health Care Management Research and Educational Foundation found a general consensus *that care should not be denied because evidence is limited, conflicting, or even non-existent.* Rather, decisions should be based on the best information available. It has been noted that:

Much, if not most, medical care, even that which is generally accepted in the medical community, would be denied under an evidence-based standard because so few health care services have been subject to rigorous research. At particular risk for denial of needed services are disabled persons because of the lack of treatments proven effective through clinical trials." (Independent Review of Managed Care Decisions by Honorable Mary C. Morgan. (Retired.)

Most patients who require prolonged intravenous antibiotics are denied coverage and subsequently undergo an independent medical review as part of the appeal process. First, it is imperative that those responsible for performing independent medical reviews be made aware of the fact that there are two recognized treatment approaches and that both sets of treatment guidelines be used as part of the review process. Second, the reviewers need to consider all of the data that illustrate the variability of treatment approaches physicians treating persistent Lyme Disease use (see Section 1 for the references). Third, the view of the treating physician needs to be given more weight, given that treatment outcomes research to date illustrate that the population being studied is enormously heterogeneous. In these situations, the clinical course of the individual patient is more a predictor of response to treatment than heterogeneous group studies. Fourth, the variation in treatment practices that currently exists should be resolved by promoting more outcomes research to help resolve the scientific uncertainty and patient's preference should be supported.

There are a number of ways that medical necessity may be determined: on facts and evidence, on a consensus of medical opinion, or on the judgment of individual physicians. Where outcomes research is limited or equivocal, decisions should be based on the best information available – which in the case of heterogeneous populations may well be the unique clinical course of the individual patient.

Section 1

Summary of Clinical Studies for Treatment of Late Stage Lyme Disease

Randomized placebo-controlled Studies

Steere, 1985[31] – 40 patients with established Lyme arthritis were randomized to receive weekly IM injections of benzathine penicillin or placebo. 35% of the treated patients had complete resolution of their symptoms and remained symptom-free during a mean follow-up period of 33 months. None of the placebo treated patients improved. As compared with nonresponders, penicillin responsive patients were more likely to have received antibiotics for early Lyme disease and less likely to have received intra-articular steroids.

Klempner, 2001[32]; Kaplan 2003[33] – 78 seropositive (by Western Blot) and 51 seronegative patients with post-treatment Lyme disease were randomized to receive 30 days IV ceftriaxone followed by oral doxycycline 100mg bid or placebo for 60 days. Patients underwent standardized testing at baseline, 90 and 180 days. *There were normal baseline neuropsychological scores in all patients.* There were no significant differences between seropositive and seronegative patients in outcomes, nor were there significant differences between treated and untreated patients. Of note is the fact that 64% of patients had persistent symptoms after standard treatment for the disease. Thus, the validity of this study has been questioned.

Krupp, 2003[34] – Double blind placebo controlled trial on 55 patients with continued fatigue 6 or more months after antibiotic treatment (3 weeks oral Abs or IV ceftriaxone) for Lyme disease. Patients were randomized to receive placebo or 4 weeks of IV ceftriaxone. Outcome measures were fatigue, cognitive speed, and clearance of OspA antigen from the CSF. 64% of patients given antibiotics were improved compared with 18.5% given placebo. Further, for patients with positive western blots at baseline, the responder rate was 80% vs 13%. For seronegative patients, the responder rate was 46% vs 27%. Patients receiving antibiotics also had significantly lower pain scores than those receiving placebo. There were no differences between groups in results of neurocognitive tests. The authors concluded that repeated antibiotic therapy had a substantial positive effect on late Lyme disease outcome.

Fallon, 2004[35] – completed a trial of 10 weeks of IV antibiotic therapy in patients with late Lyme disease symptoms who had previously been treated with at least 3 weeks of IV antibiotics and then relapsed. There was significant improvement in cognition and other symptoms. This study was part of a $4.7 million NIH funded study. The manuscript is in preparation.

Randomized Trials

<u>Dattwyler, 1988</u>[36] – 23 patients with clinically active late Lyme disease were randomly assigned to IV treatment with either penicillin or ceftriaxone. Of the 10 treated with penicillin, 5 were judged treatment failures; of the 13 who received ceftriaxone, only 1 patient did not respond. An additional 31 patients were subsequently treated with ceftriaxone with similar results. Patients that were unresponsive to ceftriaxone were more likely to have received corticosteroid treatment.

<u>Pfister, 1989</u>[37] – 21 patients with radiculitis or neuroborreliosis associated with Lyme disease were randomized to receive a 10 day treatment with either IV penicillin G or cefataxime. There were no differences in the outcomes of the two groups. See Pfister, 1991 below.

<u>Hassler, 1990</u>[38] – 135 patients with late-stage Lyme disease were randomized to receive IV penicillin G or IV cefotaxmine for 10 days. Cefotaxamine was significantly more effective than penicillin G with 87.9% vs 61.3% reporting full or partial remission of symptoms 24 months later.

<u>Pfister, 1991</u>[39] – 33 patients with Lyme neuroborreliosis were randomized to receive a 10 day course of either IV ceftriaxone or Cefotaxime. Neurologic symptoms improved or subsided in 26/30 patients-there was no difference in treatment groups. At a mean follow-up of 8 months, 17/27 patients were clini-

cally asymptomatic. Bb was isolated from the CSF of one patient 7 months after ceftriaxone therapy. Since 10 patients remained symptomatic, the authors concluded that a prolongation of therapy might be necessary.

Steere, 1994[40] – 38 patients with Lyme arthritis were randomly assigned to 30 days of treatment with either doxycycline or amoxicillin plus probenecid. Patients who had persistent arthritis 3 months following treatment were given IV ceftriaxone for 2 weeks. 16/18 of the patients treated with amoxicillin and 18/20 treated with doxycycline had resolution of arthritis symptoms within 3 months of treatment. However, neuroborreliosis later developed in 5 patients. Of 16 patients with persistent arthritis who were treated with IV ceftriaxone, none had resolution of arthritis within 3 months. The authors concluded that even with resolution of specific manifestations of Lyme disease with oral antibiotics, there is still a risk of developing additional symptoms of Lyme at a later time. Persistent arthritis may be related to an autoimmune phenomenon (although they did not rule out persistent infection with PCR or culture). Others concluded that 2 weeks of IV ceftriaxone may be insufficient to address Lyme arthritis.

Wahlberg, 1994[41] – 100 consecutive late-Lyme disease patients were treated with different antibiotic regimens and followed up for 12 months after treatment. Treatment outcome was successful in 4/13 patients treated with IV ceftriaxone for 14 days, 50/56 patients treated with ceftriaxone followed by 100 days of amoxicillin with probenecid, and 19/23 of those treated with IV ceftriaxone for 14 days followed by 100 days of cephadroxil.

Okski, 1998[42] – randomized 60 patients with disseminated Lyme borreliosis based on CDC diagnostic criteria to receive either cefexime and probenecid orally for 100 days or ceftri-axone IV for 14 days followed by oral amoxicillin and probenecid for 100 days. The immediate outcome after antibi-otics was not different between the two treatment groups. However, after a year of follow-up, there were significantly greater relapses, treatment failures, and positive PCR tests. The results of this study support the use of intravenous antibi-otics along with prolonged antibiotic therapy in patients with late-stage Lyme disease.

Fallon, 1999[43] – studied 23 Lyme patients who complained of persistent memory difficulties after IV antibiotic therapy of 4-16 weeks. Four months after their initial treatment, 18 of the patients received additional IV antibiotics and compared with the others who did not receive additional antibiotics. Those receiving additional IV antibiotics scored better on cognition tests, greatest functional improvement in energy, pain, and physical functioning than untreated patients. Based on the results from this pilot study, the authors concluded that there was enough evidence to plan a larger study investigating the utility of repeated courses of IV antibiotics (see Fallon, 2004).

Logigian, 1999[44] – a series of 18 consecutive patients with Lyme encephalopathy and symptoms of memory difficulty, minor depression, somnolence, or headache were treated with 30 days of IV ceftriaxone. At the beginning of treatment, 89% had abnormal memory scores, 89% had CSF abnormalities and all tested had perfusion defects on SPECT scan. Six months after treatment, memory scores were significantly improved, CSF protein levels were significantly less, and post-treatment perfusion was significantly improved. 12-24 months after treatment, all patients rated themselves as improved or back to normal.

Observational studies

Hassler, 1991[45] – reported on two patients with antibiotic resistant Lyme disease that were treated with pulsed high-dose cefataxime with 2 days of treatment followed by 6 days without antibiotics over a ten-week period of time. One patient was symptom-free 6 months after antibiotic treatment, the other was improved and skin biopsies showed no evidence of Borrelia.

Valesov, 1996[46] – reported on the outcome of a 36-month follow-up of patients with late stage Lyme arthritis after 2 weeks of ceftriaxone therapy. At 36 months 19/26 continued to be symptom-free, 6 had relapsed and 1 presented with new late-Lyme symptoms.

Donta, 1997[47] – 277 patients with chronic Lyme disease and symptoms of fatigue, musculoskeletal pain, neuropsychiatric dysfunction, and paresthesias were treated with tetracycline for 1-11 months (mean 4 months). Overall 20% of the patients were cured, 70% significantly improved (degree of improvement 75-100%), and 10% did not improve. Improvement frequently did not take place for several weeks: after 2 months of treatment, 33% were significantly improved, after 3 months 61% were significantly improved. Improvement showed as early as one to two weeks after the start of treatment; however, in patients who were symptomatic for more than a year, it frequently took 4-6 weeks on the antibiotic for evidence of improvement. This slow rate of improvement was postulated to be due to the slow rates of multiplication and metabolism in Borrelia. This study underscores the necessity of an individualized approach to the treatment of late-stage Lyme disease.

Okski, 1999[48] – 13 patients who had clinical relapses and were PCR positive after at least 3 months of oral antibiotics were treated with IV ceftriaxone for 4-6 weeks. None of the patients were PCR positive after treatment and 9 showed good therapeutic responses. The authors concluded that treating late Lyme disease with appropriate antibiotics for more than 3 months may not always eliminate Borrelia and that longer courses may be necessary.

Donta, 2003[49] – 235 patients with chronic Lyme disease symptoms of fatigue, musculoskeletal pain, and neurocognitive dysfunction with positive serology for Borrelia were treated with macrolide antibiotics and hydroxychloroquine for one or more months based on their level of improvement during the course of treatment. 120 patients who were improved at the discontin-uation of therapy had relapsing symptoms and were retreated with antibiotics. Of those retreated with macrolide/hydroxy-chloroquine, 32/33 had improvement, tetracycline 54/74 had improvement, IV ceftriaxone 9/23 had improvement. Thus, tetracycline and IV ceftriaxone had a much lower success rate than macrolide/hydroxychloroquine therapy.

Reviews

Cimmino, 1996[50] – reviewed the results of antibiotic treatment of Lyme arthritis in peer-reviewed journals between 1985 and 1991. The studies were small or medium-sized and not blinded. The antibiotics included Benzathine penicillin, IV penicillin G, IV ceftriaxone, IV Cefotaxime, oral doxycycline or oral amox-icillin plus Probenecid. The authors concluded that "There is no consensus on the therapeutic protocol to be adopted in Lyme arthritis. Many questions are still open about the antibiotic agents to adopt as well as the best duration of treatment."

Section 2

Relapse/Persistence of Lyme Disease Despite Antiobiotic Therapy

September 16, 2003

Straubinger, 2000[51] – [Persistence:] "Antibiotic treatment resulted in the temporary disappearance of *B. burgdorferi*

DNA. Skin samples became positive by PCR starting 60 days after treatment had ended, and additional positive samples were detected later...therapy with different antibiotics seems to reduce the load of *B. burgdorferi* infection to a level of approximately 53 to 13,078 spirochetes per 100 μg of extracted total DNA but fails to eliminate the infection." [Dogs were treated with ceftriaxone, doxycycline, or azithromycin for 30 consecutive days.] After antibiotic therapy had ended, in some treated dogs antibody titers remained at constant levels rather than decreasing further. This argues more for the persistence of the antigenic stimulus than for the complete elimination of *B. burgdorferi*." [Diagnosis:] "...DNA of heat-killed borrelia was not detectable for very long in skin tissue of an uninfected dog, implying that during natural infection the DNA of killed organisms is removed quickly and completely within a few days."

Straubinger et al, 2000[52] – 16 dogs were infected with *Borrelia burgdorferi*. 120 days after tick exposure, 12 dogs were treated with antibiotics for 30 days; 4 control dogs were not treated. "At euthanasia, single tissues of the antibiotic-treated dogs and multiple tissues of all control dogs were Borrelia-positive by polymerase chain reaction." [Persistence:] "Do the data indicate an ongoing persistent infection in these animals or only the presence of DNA remnants of dead Borrelia...? From this study and our previous investigations (20), it appears likely that *B. burgdorferi* maintains a persistent infection with live organisms albeit at a very low level." (p. 1079) [Diagnosis:] "As demonstrated by the injection of heat-killed *B. burgdor-*

feri organisms into the skin of an uninfected animal, DNA of dead organisms was detectable in our hands only for 3 weeks. These results are in concordance with a study in which persistent experimental infection with Treponema pallidum, the spirochetal agent of syphilis, was identified by PCR (21). Wicher et al. [1998] discovered that DNA of dead Treponema organisms was removed from or degraded within rabbit tissue within 15-30 days after syringe inoculation." (p. 1079) "Our studies show that at least in the dog, blood is an unreliable tissue to demonstrate *B. burgdorferi* infection." (p. 1080)

Oksi et al, 1999[53] – Of 165 patients treated for disseminated Lyme borreliosis with three months or more of antibiotics (including a minimum of two weeks of ceftriaxone), 32 had treatment failure. At follow-up, 13 patients with clinical relapse were PCR or culture positive (10 PCR positive, 1 culture positive, 2 PCR and culture positive). "In this study, culture or PCR-based evidence for the presence of live spirochetes was obtained in more than 40% of the patients with relapsed disease. The treatment caused only temporary relief in the symptoms of the patients. We conclude that the treatment of Lyme borreliosis with appropriate antibiotics for even more than 3 months may not always eradicate the spirochete."

Breier et al, 2001[54] – [From the abstract:] "Despite treatment with four courses of ceftriaxone with or without methylprednisone for up to 20 days, progression of LSA [lichen sclerosus et atrophicus] was only stopped for a maximum of 1 year.

Spirochaetes were isolated from skin cultures obtained from enlarging LSA lesions. These spirochaetes were identified as *Borrelia afzelii* by sodium sulphate-polyacrylamide gel electrophoresis and polymerase chain reaction (PCR) analyses. However, serology for *B. burgdorferi* sensu lato was repeatedly negative." [From the article:] "The relapses she repeatedly suffered despite initially successful antibiotic treatment could be related to the observation that Borrelia may possibly be able to remain dormant in certain tissue compartments, thus escaping batericidal antibiotic activity. This would be consistent with the fact that these relapses were always able to be treated successfully with a course of the same antibiotics as before; this is corroborated by a recent report that Bb may persist in experimentally infected dogs despite antibiotic treatment with doxycycline or amoxycillin."

Warner et al, 1999[55] – "Two [of three patients] had new symptoms/signs despite appropriate and adequate treatment; the third a remitting-relapsing course."

Cimperman et al, 1999[56] – [Abstract:] "The results of our study revealed that Lyme meningitis frequently occurs without meningeal signs and is often accompanied by additional borreliosis persisted or occurred for the first time in several patients. They were not infrequent even at the examination performed one year after therapy." [A total of 36 patients were followed.]

Zamponi et al, 1999[57] – [From the abstract:] "Lyme disease is a polymorphic and multisystemic disease caused by *Borrelia burgdorferi*. Neurological manifestations are found in 10%-50% of cases. We present 2 cases followed for 5 and 6 years of chronic relapsing-remitting neuroborreliosis."

Kufko et al, 1999[58] – "Patients with persistent levels of antibodies to *B. burgdorferi*, even without clinical signs of infection, are in need of regular check-ups, because the prognostic significance of antibodies to *B. burgdorferi* is unknown and relapses may occur after months and years."

Straubinger et al, 1998[59] – [Abstract:] "In three separate experiments, *B. burgdorferi*-infected dogs received antibiotic treatment (amoxicillin; azithromycin; ceftriaxone; doxycycline) for 30 consecutive days. ...Antibiotic treatment prevented or resolved episodes of acute arthritis, but failed to eliminate the bacterium from infected dogs. ...CONCLUSIONS: *B. burgdorferi* disseminates through tissue by migration following tick inoculation, produces episodes of acute arthritis, and establishes persistent infection. The spirochete survives antibiotic treatment and disease can be reactivated in immuno-suppressed animals."

Treib et al, 1998[60] – [Abstract:] "The authors performed a clinical and seriologic follow-up study after 4.2 +/- 1.2 years in 44 patients with clinical signs of neuroborreliosis and specific intrathecal antibody production. All patients had been treated with ceftriaxone 2 g/day for 10 days. Although neurologic deficits decreased significantly, more than half the patients had unspecific complaints resembling a chronic fatigue syndrome and showed persisting positive immunoglobulin M serum titers for Borrelia in the Western blot analysis."

Hudson et al, 1998[61] – "We report a case of Lyme borreliosis. Culture of skin biopsy was positive for *Borrelia garinii*, despite repeated prior treatment with antibiotics."

Meier et al, 1998[62] – "Despite of [sic] intravenous application of ceftriaxone for 14 days panuveitis persisted, and endophthalmitis developed when antibiotic therapy was finished. ...Despite a second intravenous ceftriaxone treatment for 14 days we observed a retinal vasculitis in the follow up of 6 months. CONCLUSIONS: Despite intravenous ceftriaxone-therapy *Borrelia burgdorferi* must have survived in the vitreous body."

Priem et al, 1998[63] – [Persistence:] "Paired SF [synovial fluid] and SM [synovial membrane] specimens and urine samples from four patients with ongoing or recurring Lyme arthritis despite previous antibiotic therapy were investigated. RESULTS: In all four cases, PCR with either primer set was negative in SF and urine, but was positive with at least one primer pair in the SM specimens." [Diagnosis:] "CONCLUSIONS: These data suggest that in patients with treatment resistant Lyme arthritis negative PCR results in SF after antibiotic therapy do not rule out the intraarticular persistence of *B burgdorferi* DNA. Therefore, in these patients both SF and SM should be analysed for borrelial DNA by PCR as positive results in SM are strongly suggestive of ongoing infection."

Petrovic et al, 1998[64] – A five-week treatment with doxycycline at a dose of 200 mg daily was prescribed. Fatigue, arthralgia en myalgia seemed to respond positively to the initiated therapy. However, they reappeared two weeks after cessation of doxycycline. ...it was decided to treat with ceftriaxone IM 2 g daily for three weeks. This resulted in a complete resolution of the general symptoms. However, three weeks later arthralgia of the knees and myalgia in both legs recurred. ...Symptoms and signs may improve only temporarily shortly after treatment, but re-emerge within weeks or months.

Straubinger et al, 1997[65] – [From the abstract :] "In specific-pathogen-free dogs experimentally infected with *Borrelia burgdorferi* by tick exposure, treatment with high doses of amoxicillin or doxycycline for 30 days diminished but failed to eliminate persistent infection. Although joint disease was prevented or cured in five of five amoxicillin- and five of six doxycycline-treated dogs, skin punch biopsies and multiple tissues from necropsy samples remained PCR positive and *B. burgdorferi* was isolated from one amoxicillin- and two doxycycline-treated dogs following antibiotic treatment. ...[In] dogs that were kept in isolation for 6 months after antibiotic treatment was discontinued, antibody levels began to rise again, presumably in response to proliferation of the surviving pool of spirochetes."

Straubinger et al, 1997[66] – [Persistence:] "In two studies, antibiotic treatment with amoxicillin or doxycycline for 30 days failed to eliminate persistent infection in 11 dogs. Immediately after treatment, borreliae could not be demonstrated, antibody levels declined, and joint lesions were prevented or cured. Live spirochetes, however, persisted in the tissue of at least three dogs as *B. burgdorferi* DNA was detected in all 11 treated dogs for up to 6 months after treatment, at which time antibody levels again began to rise." [Diagnostic issues:] "In the dog model, we detected *B. burgdorferi* reliably in skin but infrequently in blood by culture and polymerase chain reaction (PCR). We found the organism in the synovium of joints but not in synovial fluids, and in meninges but not in cerebrospinal fluid."

Branigan et al, 1997[67] – "PCR evidence for Borrelia has been identified in synovial biopsies of patients with clinical pictures that had not initially suggested Lyme disease. All [6 PCR-positive] patients were negative for antibodies to Borrelia and some were PCR positive in synovium despite previous treatment with antibiotics."

Weber, 1996[68] – [From the abstract:] "Patients with erythema migrans can fail to respond to antibiotic therapy. Persistent or recurrent erythema migrans, major sequelae such as meningitis and arthritis, survival of *Borrelia burgdorferi* and significant and persistent increase of antibody titres against *B. burgdorferi* after antibiotic therapy are strong indications of a treatment failure. Most, if not all, antibiotics used so far have been associated with a treatment failure in patients with erythema migrans."

Nanagara et al, 1996[69] – [From the abstract:] "Electron microscopy [both EM and IEM were used] adds further evidence for persistence of spirochetal antigens in the joint in chronic Lyme disease. Locations of spirochetes or spirochetal antigens both intracellulary and extracellulary in deep synovial connective tissue as reported here suggest sites at which spirochaetes may elude host immune response and antibiotic treatment." [From the article:] "If spirochetes are already sequestered in tissue that is inaccessible to antibiotics such as in the fibrinous and collagen tissue or within fibroblasts, high-dose parenteral antibiotics, or combination therapies with long duration may be needed to kill the living spirochetes." (p. 1032)

Mursic et al, 1996[70] – [Persistence:] "...clinical persistence of *Borrelia burgdorferi* in patients with active Lyme borreliosis occurs despite obviously adequate antibiotic therapy...The persistence of Bb even after therapy with antibiotics has been demonstrated in cerebrospinal fluid (CSF), in skin, iris, heart and joint biopsies." [Cysts:] In vitro investigation of morphological variants of *B. burgdorferi*, in an effort to explain the clinical persistence of active Lyme borreliosis despite antibiotic therapy. The authors suggest that these atypical forms may allow Borrelia to survive antibiotic treatment.

Luft et al, 1996[71] – "Fifty-seven percent of patients who had relapse were seronegative at the time of relapse."

<u>Bayer et al, 1996</u>[72] – The urine of 74.2% of patients previously treated with antibiotics for Lyme disease was found to be positive for *B. burgdorferi* DNA using PCR testing. All patients (n=97) had prior documented EM rash and had received a minimum of 3 weeks to 2 months oral or intravenous antibiotics. In 4 patients, PCR results were temporarily negative after treatment, but became positive again 4-6 weeks later. All patients suffered "continuing, often gradually worsening Lyme disease-like symptoms. ...it seems to be characteristic for most of the patients in our study that, after antibiotic-free periods of a few months, they had again become increasingly ill with neurological and arthritic symptoms, so that treatment had been resumed."

<u>Aberer et al, 1996</u>[73] – "Neuralgias arising 6 months after ECM in spite of antibiotic therapy were evident in a seronegative patient who showed perineural rod-like borrelia structures."

<u>Oksi et al, 1996</u>[74] – "In one of the six analysed brain tissue specimens [from a patient who had received more than six months of antibiotic treatment prior to death, including two 3-week courses of IV ceftriaxone], *B. burgdorferi* DNA was detected by PCR."

<u>Valesova et al, 1996</u>[75] – "Long term clinical results in 26 patients at 36 months were complete response or marked improvement in 19, relapse in six and new manifestations in four of the cases, respectively."

Preac et al, 1996[76] – [Persistence:] "...the persistence of *B. burgdorferi* s.l. and clinical recurrences in patients despite seemingly adequate antibiotic treatment is described." ...[Diagnosis:] "The patients had clinical disease with or without diagnostic antibody titers to *B. burgdorferi.*"

Lawrence et al, 1995[77] – [From the abstract:] This article reports a Lyme disease patient "who experienced repeated neurologic relapses despite aggressive antibiotic therapy." The patient was seronegative. "Although the patient never had detectable free antibodies to *B. burgdorferi* in serum or spinal fluid, the CSF was positive on multiple occasions for complexed anti-*B. burgdorferi* antibodies, *B. burgdorferi* nucleic acids and free antigen." [From the article:] "Before her 6th hospital admission this patient had received four courses of ceftriaxone, one of cefotaxime and two of doxycycline (of 19 and 8 weeks). Increasing right hemiparesis and dyspnea with right intercostal muscle weakness prompted her 6th admission to the hospital. Following intravenous ceftriaxone for 2 weeks, it was decided to place the patient on long-term therapy [22 months] with clarithromycin. Although there is no information on the penetration of clarithromycin into the CNS, it achieves high concentrations within macrophages [18] a known sanctuary for the Bb spirochete [19]. The clinical response to clarithromycin in this patient has now been sustained for over 22 months. ...Survival of Bb in humans despite aggressive antibiotic therapy has been previously reported [2,22]. We believe this to be an example of a patient with chronic relapsing Bb infection. It is important to evaluate unusual patients like this thoroughly in order to determine the effectiveness of prolonged oral antibiotics as a therapeutic option."

Waniek et al, 1995[78] – [From the abstract:] "The authors report a case of fatal neuropsychiatric Lyme disease. (LD) that was expressed clinically by progressive frontal lobe dementia and pathologically by severe subcortical degeneration. Antibiotic treatment resulted in transient improvement, but the patient relapsed after the antibiotics were discontinued. LD [Lyme disease] must be considered even in cases with purely psychiatric presentation, and prolonged antibiotic therapy may be necessary."

Steere, 1995[79] – "...a 1-month course of oral antibiotics may not always eradicate viable spirochetes."

Vartiovaara, 1995[80] – A Finnish physician's account of his experiences that beginning with a tick bite in Vancouver in 1987, Dr. Vartiovaara resigned from his position with the Finnish Medical Journal in 1992, due to disabilities caused by Lyme disease. [Persistence:] "After that [a positive result on a T-cell proliferation test at Stony Brook Hospital] I had two months' heavy treatment with oral doxycycline 300mg a day. I was a little better after it, but only for about two months. Then it started all over again, and got worse. ...We sent blood and spinal fluid to Dr. Oksi and they turned out to be positive [by PCR] – in other words, the spirochaete was still alive in my body after six years, despite the antibiotics." Dr. Varitovaara was then treated aggressively with a combination of antibiotics, including four weeks of ceftriaxone, for six months. Some time after the cessation of treatment however, he found that "My symptoms are on the move again." [Diagnosis:] "What should be done when a patient has the typical Lyme disease history but negative serology? This is still a hot question especially in the USA. My strong opinion is that oral antibiotics should be given in such cases. Ordinary laboratory tests cannot be relied upon and the PCR is too expensive for routine use. When the whole picture leans towards Lyme borreliosis it is both ethically and medically right to treat." (p. 844)

Ferris et al, 1995[81] – "Our patient received during 2 years seven short-term antibiotic treatments, achieving transitory improvements. Nonetheless, his condition greatly deteriorated. In October, 1993, he started a different antibiotic regimen (ceftriaxone, 2 g per day intravenously for 12 months, oral roxithromycin 150 mg per day for 2 months, and oral ciprofloxacin, 500 mg per 12 hours for 2 months). After ceftriaxone he has continued with oral minocycline, 100 mg per 12 hours for 7 months. His quality of life has greatly improved and the treatment is more tolerable than the borreliosis. We add however, in accord with the advice of others that antibiotics should be continued in the long term, until we achieve cure or delay the progression of the disease."

Wahlberg et al, 1994[82] – [From the abstract:] "Short periods of treatment were not generally effective." [From the article:] "Symptoms and signs often improve temporarily shortly after treatment but reappear within weeks or months. ...To conclude, we have shown that long-term treatments beginning with intravenous ceftriaxone and continuing with amoxycillin plus probenecid or with cephadroxil were useful in the treatment of late Lyme borreliosis." (pp. 260-1)

Malawista et al, 1994[83] – The mice receiving antibiotic treatment in this study were given ceftriaxone. [Persistence:] 2 out of 5 mice tested 60 days after treatment were found to be positive on culture; 1 of these mice was also positive by PCR. The authors speculate that this could be due to: (a) reinfection (which they consider "highly unlikely"), (b) contamination, or (c) the "resurgence of spirochetes in animals not completely sterilized by antibiotics. This last possibility will bear further scrutiny because late recurrences of Lyme disease without obvious reinfection may occur in humans." [Diagnosis:] Positive PCR results were found to suggest active infection. "Unless some patients with Lyme disease have a defect in their ability to degrade spirochetal DNA, these results suggest that persisting PCR positively indicates persisting infection."

Bradley et al, 1994[84] – "Our results show the intra-articular persistence of *B. burgdorferi* nucleic acids in Lyme arthritis and suggest that persistent organisms and their components are important in maintaining ongoing immune and inflammatory processes even among some antibiotic-treated patients. Further studies are needed to determine the microbiologic state of these organisms and their therapeutic and prognostic implications." (p. 489)

Asch et al, 1994[85] – [From the abstract:] "Patients were seen at a mean 3.2 years after initial treatment. A history of relapse with major organ involvement had occurred in 28% and a history of reinfection in 18%. Anti-Borrelia antibodies, initially present in all patients, were still positive in 32%. At followup, 82 (38%) patients were asymptomatic and clinically active Lyme disease was found in 19 (9%). Persistent symptoms of arthralgia, arthritis, cardiac or neurologic involvement with or without fatigue were present in 114 (53%) patients." [From the article:] "...18 patients (8%) received intravenous antibiotics (penicillin in 14 and ceftriaxone in 4) as initial therapy and 6 (33%) of these patients relapsed. ...Subsequent courses of antibiotic therapy were used in 51 (24%) patients. Many received repeated courses of antibiotic therapy for disease relapse and had full or partial response to this treatment."

Shadick et al, 1994[86] – "Ten of the 38 patients with Lyme disease reported relapses within 1 year of treatment... and had had repeated antibiotic treatment (5 patients with intravenous ceftriaxone). ...Patient 4, in addition, had had second degree atrioventricular block with acute Lyme disease that resolved with penicillin treatment. Her irregular rhythm recurred 2 years later, resolved temporarily with ceftriaxone treatment, but progressed to complete heart block requiring a pacemaker. ...Patient 12... was treated with 2 weeks of parenteral penicillin. She later developed a progressive speech disorder, bradykinesia, and abnormal ocular motor function. Magnetic resonance imaging of the brain showed scattered white matter lesions in the hemispheres and pons... she was re-treated with 2 weeks of parenteral ceftriaxone in 1989 that had no effect on her neurologic symptoms. During the time of observation, this patient died. At autopsy... [using] Dieterle silver stain, a spirochete was present in the cortex and another was exterior to a leptomeningeal vessel."

Lopez-Andreu et al, 1994[87] – "[The patient] received 2 g of ceftriaxone daily for 4 weeks. Marked early clinical improvement was observed and continued for 3 weeks after therapy was discontinued. He received 6 additional courses of intravenous antibiotics for 3 to 5 weeks' duration (penicillin, doxycycline [two courses], and ceftriaxone [three courses]), and 1 oral antibiotic (azithromycin). His general condition improved, but each antibiotic course was followed by a relapse."

Preac-Mursic et al, 1993[88] – "The persistence of *Borrelia burgdorferi* in six patients is described. *Borrelia burgdorferi* has been cultivated from iris biopsy, skin biopsy, and cerebrospinal fluid also after antibiotic therapy for Lyme borreliosis. Lyme Serology: IgG antibodies to *B. burgdorferi* were positive, IgM negative in four patients; in two patients both IgM and IgG were negative. Antibiotic therapy may abrogate the antibody response to the infection as shown by our results. Patients may have subclinical or clinical disease without diagnostic antibody titers. Persistence of *B. burgdorferi* cannot be excluded when the serum is negative for antibodies against it."

<u>Klempner et al, 1993</u>[89] – This study found that *B. burgdorferi* spirochetes can survive antibiotic treatment through intracellular sequestion within fibroblasts. "In these experiments, we demonstrated that fibroblasts and keratinocytes were able to protect *B. burgdorferi* from the action of this B-lactam antibiotic [ceftriaxone] even at antibiotic concentrations > or = 10 times the MBC of the antibiotic. The protective effect was sustained for < or = 14 days and required viable fibroblast monolayers... We have demonstrated the presence of intracellular *B. burgdorferi* within HF [human fibroblasts] using laser scanning confocal microscopy... The observation of viable spirochetes within fibroblasts coupled to protection of *B. burgdorferi* from extracellular microbicidal antibiotics by fibroblasts [19] suggests that *B. burgdorferi* may be among the small number of bacteria that can cause chronic infection by localizing within host cells where they remain sequestered from some antimicrobial agents and the host humoral immune response."

<u>Haupl et al, 1993</u>[90] – [Persistence:] "Repeated antibiotic treatment [6 weeks oral doxycycline, 2 weeks intravenous ceftriaxone, 2 weeks combination of oral roxithromycin/sulfamethoxazole/trimethoprim] was necessary to stop the progression of disease, but obviously did not completely eliminate *B. burgdorferi* from all sites of infection. This was confirmed by the culture of viable *B. burgdorferi* from a ligament sample obtained surgically. [The cultured bacteria were identified as *B. burgdorferi* by reactions with specific immune sera and monoclonal antibodies, and by polymerase chain reaction

amplification and Southern blot hybridization techniques.] ...These data indicate that vital *B. burgdorferi* persisted (a) despite several courses of antibiotic therapy, (b) even when clinical symptoms subsided, and (c) even when no humoral immune response was detectable by ELISA or by IF." (p. 1625) [Treatment:] "The hypothesis of evasion [to explain the survival of Bb] supports the use of more aggressive therapy as described in recent reports (19), in which 3-4 weeks of intravenous antibiotics was suggested as first-line treatment when systemic manifestations develop, such as the choroiditis in our patient." (p. 1626) [Intracellular:] "Electron microscopy of the ligament revealed spirochetes situated between collagen fibers or associated with fibroblasts, deeply invaginating these cells." (p. 1625) [Diagnosis:] [From the abstract:] "The initially significant immune system activation was followed by a loss of the specific humoral immune response and a decrease in the cellular immune response to *B. burgdorferi* over the course of the disease." [From the article:] "Interestingly, the cellular immune responses were also directed against the surface protein OspA during each recurrence of clinical symptoms, even though anti-OspA antibiotics were not detectable by immunoblot." (p. 1625)

Chancellor et al, 1993[91] – [From the abstract:] "Neurological and urological symptoms in all patients were slow to resolve and convalescence was protracted. Relapses of active Lyme disease and residual neurological deficits were common."

Reik, 1993[92] – [From the abstract:] "A 56-year-old Connecticut woman suffered multiple strokes 18 months after antibiotic treatment for early Lyme disease with facial palsy. Pleocytosis, intrathecal synthesis of anti-*Borrelia burgdorferi* antibody, and the response to antibiotic treatment substantiated the diagnosis of neuroborreliosis."

Battafarano et al, 1993[93] – "A patient had chronic septic Lyme arthritis of the knee for seven years despite multiple antibiotic trials and multiple arthroscopic and open synovectomies. Spirochetes were documented in synovium and synovial fluid (SF). Polymerase chain reaction (PCR) analysis of the SF was consistent with Borrelia infection."

Liu, 1993[94] – "Early cases may be cured by oral antibiotics while intravenous drip of large dosage is needed for advanced cases, with a relapsing rate of 16%.

Georgilis et al, 1992[95] – [From the abstract:] "The Lyme disease spirochete, *Borrelia burgdorferi,* can be recovered long after initial infection, even from antibiotic-treated patients, indicating that it resists eradication by host defense mechanisms and antibiotics. ...Human foreskin fibroblasts protected *B. burgdorferi* from the lethal action of a 2-day exposure to ceftriaxone at 1 microgram/mL, 10-20 x MBC. In the absense of fibroblasts, the organisms did not survive. ...Fibroblasts protected *B. burgdorferi* for at least 14 days of exposure to ceftriaxone. Mouse keratinocytes, HEp-2 cells, and Vero cells but not Caco-2 cells showed the same protective effect. Thus, several eukaryotic cell types provide the Lyme disease spirochete with a protective environment contributing to its long-term survival." [From the article:] "An intracellular site of survival would provide protection, since many of the antibiotics are much less concentrated in the cells than in extracellular spaces. ...Possibly fibroblasts and keratinocytes are the initial sites of this intracellular survival. This is especially relevant in that the first contact between the spirochete and the host in Lyme disease occurs in the skin." (p. 443)

Cooke et al, 1992[96] – "The diversity of the symptoms [of Lyme arthritis], form a mild self-limited illness to a severe chronic arthritis that persists despite antibiotic treatment, suggests that host factors are important in the pathogenesis."

Feder et al, 1992[97] – [From the abstract:] ...we recalled 32 patients with Lyme disease from a primary care practice a mean of 16 months after treatment... Nine of he 32 patients had persistent or recurrent symptoms, and ELISA and immunoblot were not helpful for identifying these nine patients."

Dinerman et al, 1992[98]– 15 patients with Lyme disease and symptoms of fibromyalgia were followed in a long-term study. "None of the patients had had fibromyalgia before the onset of Lyme disease." All patients received antibiotic therapy, in most cases 2 g/d intravenous ceftriaxone for 2 to 4 weeks. [Persistence:] "Case Report: [After 2 weeks ceftriaxone] The knee swelling gradually resolved over the next 3 months, but he [the patient] began to have symptoms of fibromyalgia including marked fatigue and more diffuse pain and stiffness in the wrists, elbows, shoulders, and knees. Because his symptoms persisted, he was given a second 2-week course of ceftriaxone 1 year later. Although his symptoms improved somewhat with treatment, his fatigue and joint pain worsened again within several months, and he also experienced intermittent headache, memory difficulties, and irritability... Because of the slight spinal fluid pleocytosis and because he had already received two courses of ceftriaxone, he was treated with imipenim, 250 mg, every 8 hours for 30 days. His symptoms again improved for several months, but then worsened. During the subsequent year, in addition to his previous symptoms, he developed radicular pain along the chest wall, numbness and sensitivity on the right side of the face, and numbness in the left hand and foot." [Diagnosis:] "None of the patients had an elevated erythrocyte sedimentation rate." [Seronegativity:] "The small percentage of patients who are seronegative by enzyme-linked immunosorbent assay (ELISA) later in the illness usually have positive Western blots or cellular immune responses to borrelial antigens (9, 10)."

Pfister et al, 1991[99] – 33 patients with Lyme neuroborreliosis were treated for 10 days with either IV ceftriaxone or IV cefotaxine. Follow-up examinations were conducted after a mean of 8.1 months. 10 of 27 patients examined were symptomatic at follow-up and borreliae persisted in the CSF of one patient.

the authors conclude that "a prolongation of therapy may be necessary."

Agger et al, 1991[100] – "Despite longer and more frequent parenteral therapy, late Lyme disease frequently required retreatment, owing to poor clinical response (p less than .05)."

MacDonald et al, 1990[101] – "Active cases of Lyme disease may show clinical relapse following antibiotic therapy. The latency and relapse phenomena suggest that the Lyme disease spirochete is capable of survival in the host for prolonged periods of time. We studied 63 patients with erythema migrans, the pathgnomonic cutaneous lesion of Lyme borreliosis, and examined in vitro cultures of biopsies from the active edge of the erythematous patch. Sixteen biopsies yielded spirochetes after prolonged incubations of up to 10.5 months, suggesting that *Borrelia burgdorferi* may be very slow to divide in certain situations. Some patients with Lyme borreliosis may require more than the currently recommended two to three week course of antibiotic therapy to eradicate strains of the spirochete which grow slowly."

Logigian et al, 1990[102] – [From the abstract:] "Six months after a two-week course of intravenous ceftriaxone (2 g daily), 17 patients (63 percent) had improvement, 6 (22 percent) had improvement but then relapsed, and 4 (15 percent) had no change in their condition." [From the article:] "Discussion... These chronic neurologic abnormalities began months to years after the onset of infection, sometimes after long periods of latency, as in neurosyphilis... The typical response of our patients to antibiotic therapy supports the role of spirochetal infection in the pathogenesis of each of the syndromes described here...The likely reason for relapse is failure to eradicate the spirochete...This is reminiscent of far advanced neurosyphilis... This last article is one of many studies that show continuing symptoms are most likely due to persistence of the spirochete."

Sigal, 1990[103] – [Relapse:] "Nine patients were seen who had a preceding history of Lyme disease and previous successful therapy, but the nonspecific symptoms had returned."

Nadelman et al, 1990[104] – [Persistent Symptoms:] "Five of seven patients remained symptomatic at a median of four months after treatment..."

Schoen, 1989[105] – [Treatment/Relapse:] "As in other spiro-chetal infections, antibiotic therapy is most effective early in the illness. ...Late Disease: Not all patients with neurologic manifestations or with arthritis respond to oral or intravenous antibiotic therapy (19), and in many of these individuals, retreatment may be necessary. Retreatment is also appropriate in individuals who relapse, for example, with recurrent arthri-tis. ...Late in the illness, cases refractory to antibiotic therapy may be encountered."

<u>Dieterle et al, 1989</u>[106] – "Despite antibiotic treatment (usually 10 mega U penicillin three times daily) six patients had a recurrence by April, 1989, treated with penicillin again or with twice daily 100 mg doxycycline or 2 g ceftriaxone."

<u>Preac-Mursic et al, 1989</u>[107] – [From the abstract:] "We conclude that early stage of the disease as well as chronic Lyme disease with persistence of *B. burgdorferi* after antibiotic therapy cannot be excluded when the serum is negative for antibodies against *B. burgdorferi*." [Persistence:] "However, some patients later developed symptoms of the disease despite antibiotic treatment (9-11). Because of these observations it has become questionable if a definite eradication of *B. burgdorferi* with antibiotics is possible." (p. 357)... "The central nervous system invasion by spirochetes and a persistence of Treponema pallidum after penicillin G therapy is common in neurosyphilis (22,23)." (p. 358) [Treatment:] "In view of the hitherto failure of treatment, low CSF concentration of penicillin G, survival of *B. burgdorferi* in patients treated with antibiotics, the moderate penicillin G susceptibility of the organism and unpredictable progression of the disease, it seems appropriate to treat patients with substantially larger doses of antibiotics and/or longer than is provided in present treatment regimens." (p. 358) [Seronegativity:] "As shown, negative antibody-titers do not provide evidence for successful therapy; antibody-titers may become negative despite persistence of *B. burgdorferi*." (p. 358)

Kohler et al, 1989[108] – [From the abstract:] "We report two cases of Lyme borreliosis (LB) with erythema migrans (EM) and simultaneous meningopolyneuritis... EM and pain disappeared completely under high-dose penicillin G therapy within a few days. Pathological findings in CSF improved. Nevertheless, during and after therapy, neurological signs of LB developed: cranial nerve palsies as well as paresis of extremity muscles with radicular distribution."

Steere et al, 1988[109] – [Persistence:] "Synovial tissue was obtained from 12 patients with Lyme disease who underwent arthroscopic synovectomy between 1984 and 1986. ...All patients had received antibiotic therapy and nonsteroidal anti-inflammatory drugs (NSAIDs) prior to arthroscopic synovectomy, (p. 488) ... "Using monoclonal antibodies to the 31- or 41-kd polypeptides of *B. burgdorferi*, a few spirochetes and globular antigen deposits were seen in and around normal or injured blood vessels in areas of lymphocytic infiltration, in 6 of the 12 patients (Figure 4)." (p. 492) "Similarly [as in tertiary syphilis or tuberculoid leprosy], the antigenic stimulus in Lyme arthritis would appear to be a small number of live spirochetes, demonstrated here by monoclonal antibodies, which may persist in the synovial lesion for years." (p. 494)

Dattwyler et al, 1988[110] – [From the abstract:] "We studied 17 patients who had presented with acute Lyme disease and received prompt treatment with oral antibiotics, but in whom chronic Lyme disease subsequently developed."

<u>Schmidli et al, 1988</u>[111] – "Despite clinical resolution of paralysis, subsequent arthritic complication occurred. To our knowledge, this is the first report of the successful isolation of *B. burgdorferi* from synovial fluid and the subsequent propagation through serial passage. This positive culture strongly suggests that the spirochetes were not eradicated by the initial antimicrobial regimens [12 days amoxicillin-clavulanate followed by two weeks of doxycycline, 200 mg/d]. ...Other possible explanations of treatment failure, such as insufficient patient compliance or reinfection by *B. burgdorferi,* were excluded by close medical and parental supervision." The patient was subsequently treated with 14 days intravenous ceftriaxone. Her arthritic symptoms resolved, and she remained symptom-free during an 11-month follow-up period.

<u>Berger, 1988</u>[112] – "Two of 80 patients with a minor form of the illness and 17 of 81 patients with a major form of the illness required retreatment."

<u>Weber et al, 1988</u>[113] – "We now demonstrate *B. burgdorferi* in the brain and liver of a newborn whose mother had been treated with oral penicillin for LB [Lyme borreliosis] during the first trimester of pregnancy. ...The death of the newborn was probably due to a respiratory failure as a consequence of perinatal brain damage."

<u>Dattwyler et al, 1987</u>[114] – "We describe the clinical courses of 5 patients with Lyme disease who developed significant late

complications, despite receiving tetracycline early in the course of their illness. All 5 patients had been treated for erythema chronicum migrans with a course of tetracycline that met or exceeded current recommendations.

Berger, 1986[115] – "Fourteen of sixty-one patients with a major form of the illness required retreatment, and five developed posttreatment late manifestations of Lyme disease consisting of Bell's palsy and persistent joint pain."

Steere et al, 1983[116] – [From the abstract:] "However, with all three antibiotic agents nearly half of the patients had minor late symptoms such as headache, musculoskeletal pain, and lethargy. These complications correlated significantly with the initial severity of illness."

Steere et al, 1977[117] – "We remain skeptical that antibiotic therapy helps... Eight of our patients received penicillin, erythromycin, or cephalexin before entering the study because of he skin lesion. In one of them, the lesion persisted for 2 months despite therapy, longer than in any of the other study patients, and seven of the eight patients still developed joint, neurologic, or cardiac abnormalities."

Halperin et al, 1992[118] – "Particularly puzzling has been the observation that organisms are extremely difficult to find in infected tissue, using either microbiologic or morphologic techniques. However, in many instances continued infection appears to be essential for symptoms to persist, no matter how small the number of organisms, as antimicrobial therapy is generally followed by clinical improvement."

1.   Jacobs, RA. Infectious Diseases: Spirochetal. Current Medical Diagnosis and Treatment (Lange Medical Books/McGraw-Hill, NY, 39th edition, 2000.

2.   Donta ST. Tetracycline therapy for chronic Lyme disease. Clin Infect Dis 1997; Suppl 1:S52-S56.

3.   United States of America Department of Health and Hyman Services Food and Drug Administration Center for Biologics Evaluation and Research Vaccines and Related Biological products Advisory Committee Meeting, May 26, 1998.

4.   Benach JL, Coleman JL, Habicht GS: Serologic evidence for simultaneous occurrences of Lyme disease and babesiosis. J Infect Dis 144:473-477, 1981.

5.   Preac-Mursic V, et al. Formation and Cultivation of *Borrelia burgdorferi* Spheroblast-L Form Variants. Infection 24(1996);3.

6.   Klempner et al. Invasion of Human Skin Fibroblasts by the Lyme Disease Spirochete, *Borrelia burgdorferi*. J Infect Diseases 1993;67:1074-81.

7.   Ma et al. Intracellular localization of *Borrelia burgdorferi* within human endothelial cells. Infect Immun 1991;59:671-78.

8.   Duray PH, Johnson RC. The histopathology of experimentally infected hamsters with the Lyme disease spirochete, *Borrelia burgdorferi*. Proc Soc Exp Biol Med. 1986: 263-269.

9.   Georgilis et al. Fibroblasts Protect the Lyme Spirochete, *Borrelia burgdorferi*, from Ceftriaxone in vitro. J. Infec. Dis. 1992:166:440-4.

10. Jaruratanasirkul et al. Distribution of Azithromycin into brain tissue, cerebrospinal fluid, and aqueous humor of the eye. Anti Agents Chemo 40:825-26, 1996.

11. Chopra et al. Tetracycline antibiotics: mode of action, applications, molecular biology, and epidemiology of bacterial resistance. Microbiol Mol Biol Rev 65: 232-60, 2001.

12. Klempner et al. Two controlled trials of antibiotic treatment in patients with persistent symptoms and a history of Lyme disease. N Engl J Med 345:85-92, 2001.

13. Asch et al. Lyme disease: An infectious and postinfectious syndrome. J Rheum 21:454-60, 1994.

14. Valesov et al. Long-term results in patients with Lyme arthritis following treatment with ceftriaxone. Infec 24:98-102, 1996.

15. Steere et al. Treatment of Lyme arthritis. Arth Rheum 37:878-88, 1994.

16. Schmidli et al. Cultivation of *Borrelia burgdorferi* from joint fluid three months after treatment of facial palsy due to Lyme

borreliosis. J Infect Dis 1988;158:905-6.

17.   Haupl, et al. Persistence of B. burgdorferi in Ligamentous Tissue from a Patient with Chronic Lyme Borreliosis. Arthritis Rheum 1993; 36:1621-6.

18.   Pfister et al. Randomized comparison of ceftriaxone and cefotaxime in Lyme neuroborreliosis. J Infect Dis. 1991; 163(2): 311-318.

19.   Hassler et al. Pulsed High Dose Cefotaxime Therapy in Refractory Lyme Borreliosis (Letter) Lancet; 338:193.

20.   MacDonald et al. Clinical implications of delayed growth of the Lyme borreliosis spirochete, *Borrelia burgdorferi*. Acta Tropica 1991;48:89-94.

21.   Wormser, et al., Practice guidelines for the treatment of Lyme disease. The Infectious Diseases Society of America. Clin Infect Dis, 2000. 31 Suppl 1: p. 1-14.

22.   The International Lyme and Associated Diseases Society (ILADS), Evidence-based guidelines for the management of Lyme disease. Expert Rev Anti-infect Ther, 2004. 2(Suppl): p. S1-S13.

23.   Jones, JH. Bad Blood: The Tuskegee Syphilis Experiment, expanded edition (New York: Free Press, 1993).

24.   Hurwitz, B., Clinical guidelines and the law. BMJ, 1995. 311: p. 1517-1518.

25.   Ziska, et al. Physician preferences in the diagnosis and treatment of Lyme disease in the United States. Infection, 1996. 24(2): p. 182-6.

26.   Fallon, B.A., Testimony at public hearings in re Lyme disease for the State of Connecticut Department of Public Health. 2004: p. 134-153.

27.   Katzel, J., Is there a consensus in treatment of Lyme Borreliosis?, in Lyme Disease 1991 Patient/Physician Perspectives from the U.S. & Canada, L. Mermin, Editor. 1992.

28.   American Medical Association, Code of Medical Ethics.

29.   Hitt, J., The year in ideas: a to z.; evidence-based medicine, in New York Times (December 9, 2001, Sunday).

30.   Wennberg, et al. Geography and the debate over Medicare reform. Health Aff (Millwood), 2002. Supp Web Exclusives: p. W96-114.

31.   Steere et al. Successful parenteral penicillin therapy of established Lyme arthritis. N Engl J Med 312:869-74, 1985.

32.   Klempner et al, Two controlled trials of antibiotic treatment in patients with persistent symptoms and a history of Lyme disease. N Engl J Med 345:85-92, 2001.

33.   Kaplan et al, Cognitive function in post-treatment Lyme disease: Do additional antibiotics help? Neurology 60:1916-1922, 2003.

34.   Krupp et al. Study and treatment of post Lyme disease. A randomized double masked clinical trial. Neurology 60(12):1923-30.

35.   In preparation.

36.   Dattwyler et al. Treatment of late Lyme borreliosis-randomized comparison of ceftriaxone and penicillin. Lancet, May 28: 1191-4, 1988.

37.   Pfister et al. Cefotaxime vs penicillin F for acute neurologic manifestations in Lyme borreliosis. A prospective randomized study. Arch Neurol 46:1190-4, 1989.

38.   Hassler et al. Cefotaxime versus penicillin in the late stage of Lyme disease-prospective, randomized therapeutic trial. Infection 18:16-20, 1990.

39.   Pfister et al. Randomized comparison of ceftriaxone and cefotaxime in Lyme neuroborreliosis. J Infect Dis 163:311-18, 1991.

40.   Steere et al. Treatment of Lyme arthritis. Arthritis Rheum 37:878-88, 1994.

41.   Wahlberg et al. Treatment of late Lyme borreliosis. J Infec 29:255-61, 1994.

42.   Oski, et al. Comparison of oral cefixime and intravenous ceftriaxone followed by oral amoxicillin in disseminated Lyme borreliosis. Eur J Clin Microbiol Infec Dis 17:715-19, 1998.

43.   Fallon et al. Repeated antibiotic treatment in chronic Lyme dis-

ease. J Spirochetal Tick Dis 6:94-101, 1999.

44.   Logigian et al. Successful treatment of Lyme encephalopathy
       with intravenous ceftriaxone. J Infec Dis 180:377-83, 1999.

45.   Hassler et al. Pulsed high-dose cefotaxime therapy in refractory
       Lyme borreliosis. The Lancet 338:1991.

46.   Valesov et al. Long-term results in patients with Lyme arthritis
       following treatment with ceftriaxone. Infection 24:98-102,
       1996.

47.   Donta ST. Tetracycline therapy for chronic Lyme disease. Clin
       Infect Dis 1997; Suppl 1:S52-S56.

48.   Oksi et al. *Borrelia burgdorferi* detected by culture and PCR in
       clinical relapse of disseminated Lyme borreliosis. Annals of
       Medicine 31: 225-32, 1999.

49.   Donta ST. Macrolide therapy of chronic Lyme disease. Med Sci
       Monit 9:136-142, 2003.

50.   Cimmino et al. Treatment of Lyme arthritis. Infection 1:91-94,
       1996.

51.   Straubinger RK. PCR-based quantification of *Borrelia burgdor-
       feri* organisms in canine tissues over a 500-day postinfection
       period. Journal of Clinical Microbiology, 2000.   38(6):2191-
       2199.

52.   Straubinger RK, Straubinger AF, Summers BA, Jacobson RH.
       Status of *Borrelia burgdorferi* Infection after antibiotic treatment

and the effects of corticosteroids: an experimental study. Journal of Infectious Diseases, 2000. 181(3):1069-1081.

53.   Oksi J, Marjamaki M, Nikoskelainen J, Viljanen MK. *Borrelia burgdorferi* detected by culture and PCR in clinical relapse of disseminated Lyme Borreliosis. 1999. Annals of Medicine, 31(3): 225-32.

54.   Breier F, Khanakah G, Stanek G, Kunz G, Aberer E, et al. Isolation and polymerase chain reaction typing of *Borrelia afzelii* from a skin lesion in a seronegative patient wtih generalized ulcerating bullous lichen sclerosus et atrophicus. 2001. Br J Dermatol, 144(2):387-392.

55.   Warner G, O'Connell S, Lawton N. Atypical features in three patients with florid neurological Lyme disease. 1999. J Neurol Neurosurg Psychiatry, 67(2):275.

56.   Cimperman J, Maraspin V, Lotric-Furlan S, Ruzic-Sabljic E, Strle F. Lyme meningitis: a one-year follow up controlled study. 1999. Wien Klin Wochenschr, 111(22-23):961-3.

57.   Zamponi N, Cardinali C, Tavoni MA, Porfiri L, Rossi R, Manca A. Chronic neuroborreliosis in infancy. 1999. Ital J Neurol Sci, Oct;20(5):303-7.

58.   Kufko IT, Mel'nikov VG, Andreeva EA, Sokolova ZI, Lesniak OM, Beikin IaB. Comparative study of results of serological diagnosis of Lyme borreliosis by indirect immunofluorescence and immunoenzyme analysis. 1999. Klin Lab Diagn, 3:34-7.

59.   Straubinger RK, Straubinger AF, Summers BA, Jacobson RH,

Erb HN. Clinical manifestations, pathogenesis, and effect of antibiotic treatment on Lyme borreliosis in dogs. 1998. Wien Klin Wochenschr, 110(24):874-81.

60.   Treib J, Fernandez A, Haass A, Grauer MT, Holzer G, Woessner R. Clinical and serologic follow-up in patients with neuroborreliosis. 1998. Neurology, Nov;51(5):1489-91.

61.   Hudson BJ, Stewart M, Lennox VA, Fukunaga M, Yabuki M, et al. Culture-positive Lyme borreliosis. 1998. Med J Aust, May 18;168(10):500-2.

62.   Meier P, Blatz R, Gau M, Spencker FB, Wiedemann P. Pars plana vitrectomy in *Borrelia burgdorferi* endophthalmitis. 1998. Klin Monatsbl Augenheilkd, 213(6):351-4.

63.   Priem S, Burmester GR, Kamradt T, Wolbart K, Rittig MG, Krause A. Detection of *Borrelia burgdorferi* by polymerase chain reaction in synovial membrane, but not in synovial fluid from patients with persisting Lyme arthritis after antibiotic therapy. 1998. Annals of the Rheumatic Diseases, 57(2):118-21.

64.   Petrovic M, Vogelaers D, Van Renterghern L, Carton D, et al. Lyme borreliosis - A review of the late stages and treatment of four cases. 1998. Acta Clinica Belgica, 53(3):178-83.

65.   Straubinger RK, Summers BA, Chang YF, Appel MJ. Persistence of *Borrelia burgdorferi* in experimentally infected dogs after antibiotic treatment. 1997. Journal of Clinical Microbiology, 35(1):111-6.

66. Straubinger RK, Straubinger AF, Jacobson RH, Chang Y, Summer BA, Hollis N, Appel M. Two lessons from the canine model of Lyme Disease: migration of *Borrelia burgdorferi* in tissues and persistence after antibiotic treatment. 1997. Journal of Spirochetal & Tick-borne Diseases, Vol. 4, No. 1/2.

67. Branigan P, Rao J, Rao J, Gerard H, Hudson A, Williams W, Arayssi T, Pando J, Bayer M, Rothfuss S, Clayburne G, Sieck M, Schumacher HR. PCR evidence for *Borrelia burgdorferi* DNA in synovium in absence of positive serology. 1997. American College of Rheumatology, Vol 40(9) Suppl. Sept, p.S270.

68. Weber K. Treatment failure in erythema migrans: a review. 1996. Infection, 24:73-5.

69. Nanagara R, Duray PH, Schumacher HR Jr. Ultrastructural demonstration of spirochetal antigens in synovial fluid and synovial membrane in chronic Lyme disease: possible factors contributing to persistence of organisms. 1996. Human Pathology, Vol 27(10); 1025-34.

70. Mursic VP, Wanner G, Reinhardt S, Wilske B, Busch U, Marget W. Formation and cultivation of *Borrelia burgdorferi* spheroplast L-form variants. 1996. Infection, 24(3):218-26.

71. Luft BJ, Dattwyler RJ, Johnson RC, Luger SW, Bosler EM, Rahn DW, et al. Azithromycin compared with amoxicillin in the treatment of erythema migrans. A double-blind, randomized, controlled trial. 1996. Annals of Internal Medicine, 124(9):785-91.

72.   Bayer ME, Zhang L, Bayer MH. *Borrelia burgdorferi* DNA in the urine of treated patients with chronic Lyme disease symptoms. A PCR study of 97 cases. 1996. Infection, 24 No. 5.

73.   Aberer E, Kersten A, Klade H, Poitschek C, Jurecka W. Heterogeneity of *Borrelia burgdorferi* in the skin. 1996. American Journal of Dermatopathology, 18(6):571-9.

74.   Oksi J, Kalimo H, Marttila RJ, Marjamaki M, Sonninen P, et al. Inflammatory brain changes in Lyme borreliosis. A report on three patients and review of literature. 1996. Brain, Dec;119 (Pt 6):2143-54.

75.   Valesova H, Mailer J, Havlik J, Hulinska D, Hercogova J. Long-term results in patients with Lyme arthritis following treatment with ceftriaxone. 1996. Infection, 24(1):98-102.

76.   Preac Mursic V, Marget W, Busch U, Pleterski Rigler D, Hagl S. Kill kinetics of *Borrelia burgdorferi* and bacterial findings in relation to the treatment of Lyme borreliosis. 1996. Infection, 24(1):9-16.

77.   Lawrence C, Lipton RB, Lowy FD, Coyle PK. Seronegative chronic relapsing neuroborreliosis. 1995. European Neurology, 35(2):113-7.

78.   Waniek C, Prohovnik I, Kaufman MA, Dwork AJ. Rapidly progressive frontal-type dementia associated with Lyme disease. 1995. Journal of Neuropsychiatry Clin Neurosci, 7(3):345-7.

79. Steere AC. Musculoskeletal manifestations of Lyme disease. 1995. American Journal of Medicine, 88:4A-44S-51S.

80. Vartiovaara I. Living with Lyme. 1995. Lancet, 345:842-4.

81. Ferris J, Lopez-Andreu JA, Salcede-Vivo J, Sala-Lizarraga JA. Lyme borreliosis. [Letter]. 1995. Lancet, Vol 345:1436-37.

82. Wahlberg P, Granlund H, Nyman D, Panelius J, Seppala I. Treatment of Lyme borreliosis. 1994. Journal of Infection, 3:255-61.

83. Malawista SE, Barthold SW, Persing DH. Fate of *Borrelia burgdorferi* DNA in tissues of infected mice after antibiotic treatment. 1994. Journal of Infectious Diseases, 170:1312-1316.

84. Bradley JF, Johnson RC, Goodman JL. The persistence of spiro-chetal nucleic acids in active Lyme arthritis. 1994. Annals of Internal Medicine, 120(6):487-9.

85. Asch ES, Bujak DI, Weiss M, Peterson MG, Weinstein A. Lyme disease: an infectious and postinfectious syndrome. 1994. Journal of Rheumatology, 3:454-61.

86. Shadick NA, Phillips CB, Logigian EL, Steere AC, Kaplan RF, Berardi AB, Duray PH, Larson MG, Wright EA, Ginsburg KS, Katz JN, Liang MH. The long-term clinical outcomes of Lyme disease. A population-based retrospective cohort study. 1994. Annals of Internal Medicine, 121(8):560-7.

87.   Lopez-Andreu JA, Ferris J, Canosa CA, Sala-Lizarraga JA. Treatment of late Lyme disease: a challenge to accept. 1994. Journal of Clinical Microbiology, 32:1415-16.

88.   Preac-Mursic V, Pfister HW, Spiegel H, Burk R, Wilske B, Reinhardt S, Bohmer R. First isolation of *Borrelia burgdorferi* from an iris biopsy. 1993. Journal of Clinical Neuro-ophthalmology, Sep;13(3):155-61; discussion 162.

89.   Klempner MS, Noring R, Rogers RA. Invasion of human skin fibroblasts by the Lyme disease spirochetes, *Borrelia burgdorferi*. 1993. Journal of Infectious Diseases, 167:1074-1081.

90.   Haupl T, Hahn G, Rittig M, Krause A, Schoerner C, Schonherr U, Kalden JR, Burmester GR. Persistence of *Borrelia burgdorferi* in ligamentous tissue from a patient with chronic Lyme borreliosis. 1993. Arthritis & Rheumatism, 36(11);1621-6.

91.   Chancellor MB, McGinnis DE, Shenot PJ, Kiilholma P, Hirsch IH. Urinary dysfunction in Lyme disease. 1993. Journal of Urology, Jan;149(1):26-30.

92.   Reik L Jr. Stroke due to Lyme disease. 1993. Neurology, 43(12):2705-7.

93.   Battafarano DF, Combs JA, Enzenauer RJ, Fitzpatrick JE. Chronic septic arthritis caused by *Borrelia burgdorferi*. 1993. Clinical Orthop, 297:238-41.

94.   Liu AN. Lyme disease in China and its ocular manifestations.

1993. Chung Hua Yen Ko Tsa Chih, 5:271-3.

95.   Georgilis K, Peacocke M, Klempner MS. Fibroblasts protect the Lyme disease spirochete, *Borrelia burgdorferi*, from ceftriaxone in vitro. 1992. Journal of Infectious Diseases, 166(2):440-4.

96.   Cooke WD, Dattwyler RJ. Complications of Lyme borreliosis. 1992. Annual Review of Medicine, 43:93-103.

97.   Feder HM Jr, Gerber MA, Luger SW, Ryan RW. Persistence of serum antibodies to *Borrelia burgdorferi* in patients treated for Lyme disease. 1992. Clinical Infectious Diseases, Nov;15(5):788-93.

98.   Dinerman H, Steere AC. Lyme disease associated with fibromyalgia. 1992. Annals of Internal Medicine, 117:281-5.

99.   Pfister HW, Preac-Mursic V, Wilske B, Schielke E, Sorgel F, Einhaupl KM. Randomized comparison of ceftriaxone and cefotaxime in Lyme neuroborreliosis. 1991. Journal of Infectious Diseases, Feb;163(2):311-8.

100.   Agger W. Case KL, Bryant GL, Callister SM. Lyme disease: clinical features, classification, and epidemiology in the upper midwest. 1991. Medicine (Baltimore) Mar;70(2):83-90.

101.   MacDonald AB, Berger BW, Schwan TG. Clinical implications of delayed growth of the Lyme borreliosis spirochete, *Borrelia burgdorferi*. 1990. Acta Trop, Dec;48(2):89-94.

102. Logigian EL, Kaplan RF, Steere AC. Chronic neurologic manifestations of Lyme disease. 1990. New England Journal of Medicine. Nov 22; 323(21):1438-44.

103. Sigal LH. Summary of the first 100 patients seen at a Lyme disease referral center. 1990. American Journal of Medicine, 88:577-581.

104. Nadelman RB, Pavia CS, Magnarelli LA, Wormser GP. Isolation of *Borrelia burgdorferi* from the blood of seven patients with Lyme disease. 1990. American Journal of Medicine, 88:21-26.

105. Schoen RT. Treatment of Lyme disease. 1989. Connecticut Medicine, Vol 53(6):335-337.

106. Dieterle L, Kubina FG, Staudacher T, Budingen HJ. Neuro-borreliosis or intervertebral disk prolapse? 1989. Dtsch Med Wochenschr, 114(42);1602-6.

107. Preac-Mursic V, Weber K, Pfister HW, Wilske B, et al. Survival of *Borrelia burgdorferi* in antibiotically treated patients with Lyme borreliosis. 1989. Infection, 17(6):355-9.

108. Kohler J, Schneider H, Vogt A. High-dose intravenous penicillin G does not prevent further progression in early neurological manifestation of Lyme borreliosis. 1989. Infection, 17(4):216-7.

109. Steere AC, Duray PH, Butcher EC. Spirochetal antigens and lymphoid cell surface markers in Lyme synovium and tonsillar

lymphoid tissue. 1988. Arthritis & Rheumatism, 31:487-495.

110. Dattwyler RJ, Volkman DJ, Luft BJ, Halperin JJ, Thomas J, Golightly MG. Seronegative Lyme disease. Dissociation of specific T- and B-lymphocyte responses to *Borrelia burgdorferi*. 1988. New England Journal of Medicine, 319(22):1441-6.

111. Schmidli J, Hunziker T, Moesli P, et al. Cultivation of *Borrelia burgdorferi* from joint fluid three months after treatment of facial palsy due to Lyme borreliosis. 1988. Journal of Infectious Diseases, 158:905-906.

112. Berger BW. Treatment of erythema chronicum migrans of Lyme disease. 1988. Annals of the New York Academy of Sciences, 539:346-51.

113. Weber K, Bratzke HJ, Neubert U, Wilske B, Duray PH. *Borrelia burgdorferi* in a newborn despite oral penicillin for Lyme borreliosis during pregnancy. 1988. Pediatric Infectious Disease Journal, 7:286-9.

114. Dattwyler RJ, Halperin JJ. Failure of tetracycline therapy in early Lyme disease. 1987. Arthritis & Rheumatism, 30:448-450.

115. Berger BW. Treating erythema chronicum migrans of Lyme disease. 1986. Journal of Am Acad Dermatology, Sep;15(3):459-63.

116. Steere AC, Hutchinson GJ, Rahn DW, Sigal LH, Craft JE, DeSanna ET, Malawista SE. Treatment of the early manifesta-

tions of Lyme disease. 1983. Annals of Internal Medicine, Jul;99(1):22-6.

117.   Steere AC, Malawista SE, Hardin JA, Ruddy S, Askenase PW, Andiman WA. Erythema chronicum migrans anad Lyme arthritis. The enlarging clinical spectrum. 1977. Annals of Internal Medicine, 86:685-698.

118.   Halperin, JJ, Heyes MP. Neuroactive kynurenines in Lyme borreliosis. 1992. Neurology, (42):43-50.

Posted with written permission and my thanks to:
Deborah A. Metzger, PhD, MD
Harmony Women's Health
851 Fremont Ave., Suite 104
Los Altos, CA 94024
650-229-1010
www.harmonywomenshealth.com

APPENDIX E
False Negative Lyme Tests

Dr. Robert Bransfield is a brilliant physician from New Jersey who sees many individuals with Tick-borne illness, since his state has a large number of infected deer ticks that are close to people. He kindly has taken the time to list all the major reasons that an individual can be infected with Lyme (and Babesia)—sometimes obviously ill with Tick-borne infections or with a clear Lyme rash—and still have negative results on common lab tests. To understand his list, you should understand that immune complexes are antibodies bound to parts of the Lyme bacteria or Babesia parasite. Lyme bacteria come in many forms such as spirochetes, blebs or dormant L-forms. You should also understand that an "antigen" is merely a fancy word for a part of the infectious agent.

If you do not understand every word below, your physician should. But at least you will understand the basic ELISA or IgG and IgM antibody tests are not reliable at detecting Lyme. This is applicable to Babesia because many of the same problems with Lyme testing apply to Babesia testing. **And if you have a negative test for Lyme, most physicians will never consider a Babesia infection.**

Why Can I Have Lyme
But My Lyme Test Results are Negative

1. Recent infection before immune response

2. Antibodies are in immune complexes

3. Spirochete encapsulated by host tissue (i.e. lymphocytic cell walls)

4. Spirochete is deep in host tissue (i.e. fibroblasts, neurons, etc.)

5. Blebs in body fluid, no whole organisms needed for PCR

6. No spirochetes in body fluid on day of test

7. Genetic heterogeneity (300 strains, 100 in U.S.)

8. Antigenic variability

9. Surface antigens change with temperature

10. Utilization of host protease instead of microbial protease

11. Spirochete in dormancy phase (L-form) with no cell walls

12. Recent antibiotic treatment

13. Recent anti-inflammatory treatment

14. Concomitant infection with Babesia may cause immuno-suppression

15. Other causes of immunosuppression

16. Lab with poor technical capability for Lyme disease

17. Lab tests not standardized for late stage disease

18. Lab tests labeled "for investigational use only"

19. CDC criteria is epidemiological not a diagnostic criteria (They set the bar for diagnosis very high to avoid any false positives, but this bar is good only for careful research or trend monitoring, and is not meant to be used clinically where these criteria will miss positive patients – JS.)

20. Lack of standardized control

21. Most controls use only a few strains as reference point

22. Few organisms are sometimes present

23. Encapsulated by glycoprotein "S-layer" which impairs immune recognition

24. "S"- layer binds to IgM

25 Immune deficiency

26. Possible down regulation of immune system by cytokines

27. Revised Western Blot criteria fails to include most significant antigens. (Some of the most specific and important Lyme proteins are missing from large national lab Western Blot tests. Or the number of specific Lyme proteins tested for is only a mere two proteins – JS.)

Slightly modified from an article by:
Robert C. Bransfield, MD
http://www.mentalhealthandillness.com

APPENDIX F

Artemisia and Its Derivatives

Informed Consent

1) I understand that the FDA approves no form of Artemisia for medical purposes. The FDA has **not approved** any herbal medicines for the treatment or cure of any disease or illness.

2) I understand that I have other options for treatment and I insist on this option.

3) I understand it is suggested that I seek other medical opinions to determine if I have Babesia or malaria. I must have at least one other evaluation if it is possible I have malaria, Babesia or cancer. I can always freely seek other opinions about the use of Artemisia derivatives.

4) I understand that in the USA, Babesia is believed to generally be a very rare illness by most physicians and health departments, and therefore it is not routinely tested for in individuals with Lyme or deer tick bites or deer tick exposure.

5) I understand that no one is able to routinely diagnose all the possible forms of Babesia in the USA. So it is possible I could be treated for an infection I do not have, i.e., Babesia.

6) I understand some studies suggest Artemisia derivatives

may harm hearing and/or hurt the brain.

7) I agree never to increase or double my dose.

8) I understand I have the option of NOT using Artemisia-related treatment to treat possible Babesia. Indeed, I am the one who is going to seek out this treatment and purchase this class of herbs myself.

9) I understand I can stop this herbal medicine at any time.

10) I understand that most infection experts, internists and family doctors do not believe Babesia is common in any location in the United States, and would typically oppose both the diagnosis of Babesia and any treatment with Artemisia products. Further, no cancer centers in the United States routinely prescribe Artemisia products for any form of cancer.

11) The possible interactions with this herb are unclear. I feel that injury or illness resulting from this herb or its interactions should not be blamed on my physician. I understand that the liver has various enzymes to remove drugs. I understand that artemisinin increases or induces CYP3A4 enzymes, profoundly inhibits CYP1A2, and creates many CYP2B6 enzymes. I can read about these groups of medications at: http://medicine.iupui.edu/flockhart/table.htm. Yet I understand data on interactions with Artemisia and its derivatives is very preliminary.

12) I understand my physician will not terminate me just because I refuse to take this herbal medication.

13) I agree not to bring any malpractice suits against any health care provider suggesting this treatment to me, nor to defame the good name of this health care provider who is trying to help me. I will not defame him or her to friends, relatives or government officers or agencies. My use of this treatment is entirely my own decision.

14) I take full responsibility for this treatment and no one is forcing me to take this herbal medicine or any of my other treatments.

15) My health care provider does NOT claim to be an expert in the use of Artemisia or its derivatives.

16) My health care provider does not claim to be an expert in the diagnosis or treatment of Babesia or malaria.

17) I understand Artemisia is NOT the standard of care or promoted by ANY cancer society in the United States.

18) My health care provider cannot guarantee the purity, potency or safety of any herb or medication. This is the responsibility of third party suppliers, and not my health care provider(s).

Artemisia and Its Derivatives
Informed Consent

Patient Name Printed   _____

Patient Name Signed _____

Patient Date of Birth   _____

Date of Signature   _____

IF I DO NOT HAVE TIME TO FULLY REFLECT ON THIS CONSENT, I WILL READ IT *FULLY* BEFORE I PURCHASE OR TAKE ANY HERBAL PRODUCT OF ANY KIND.

☙

Informed Consent Disclaimer

The medical ideas, health thoughts, health comments, products and any claims made about specific illnesses, diseases, and causes of health problems in this book, have not been evaluated by the FDA, the USDA, OSHA, CDC, NIH, NIMH, IDSA or the AMA. Never assume any United States medical body or society, or the majority of American physicians endorse any comment in this book. No comment in this book is approved by any government agency, medical body or medical society. Nothing in this book is to be used to diagnose, treat, cure or prevent disease. The information provided in this book is for educational purposes only and is not intended as a substitute for the advice from your physician or other health care professional. This book is not intended to replace or adjust any information contained on or in any product label or packaging.

You should not use the information in this book for diagnosis or treatment of any health problem, or for prescription of any medication or other treatment. You should consult with a health care professional before deciding on any diagnosis, or initiating any treatment plan of any kind. Dr. Schaller does not claim to be an expert in any illness, disease or treatment. In this book, he is merely sharing one of his interests. Please do not start any diet, exercise or supplementation program, or take any type of nutrient, herb, or medication without clear consultation with your licensed health care provider.

APPENDIX G

Additional Liver Nutrition Information

Earlier in this book I tried to focus on the most critical parts of liver health and detoxification. Yet for those with an interest, here are some other nutrients that would increase your liver health and the ability to remove various toxins. As a rule, any good routine supplement should have most of these ingredients. As you read below, you will see the liver benefits from a wide range of amino acids, vitamins and minerals. Even some enzymes are helpful in catching excess free radicals.

To start off this additional liver information appendix, here are amino acids used in the Phase II liver detox pathway: glycine, cysteine, glutamine, methionine, taurine, glutamic acid and aspartic acid.

Further, every liver cell makes energy. It makes the energy in the furnace of the cell – the mitochondria. When we make energy, sparks fly out of the mitochondria and slowly cause disease, like wet wood placed in a fireplace. The wood makes a popping sound as the water in the wood expands and blows off bits of flaming wood.

Antioxidants catch flying particles that damage tissue – including the liver. Do not expect the damage to show up in routine Liver Function Tests.

Examples of some anti-oxidants in some supplements:
• Superoxide dismutase – an enzyme that catches sparks which has been shown to increase animal and bug life spans.

- Beta-carotene and other carotenoids from supplements or foods (broccoli, spinach, yellow squash, sweet potato).

- Vitamin E – natural is best and get a form that includes many forms not just cheap "alpha."

- Vitamin C – 1,000 mg a day is good. If you are a smoker you lose about 1,000 mg every day, and so you would probably need higher amounts. The best form may be Ester C and it is highly absorbed.

- Selenium – the best form is likely L-Methionine and 200 micrograms is a common dose. Few American farms have large amounts of selenium in their soil, so adding a supplement is wise.

Other Nutrients Help Liver Enzymes Work

- B vitamins like riboflavin and niacin

- Magnesium

- Iron – women and children often do well on just the right amount. If a woman has a heavy period or bleeds over six days, this should be investigated because too much iron is being lost. Children increase their number of red blood cells as they grow and require iron to fill these new red blood cells. But too much iron increases sparking free radicals. So review the best dosing for your gender and age with a nutrition expert. We suggest animal-based heme ferrous iron because it is absorbed much better than other forms. It also seems to have less stomach and intestinal side effects.

- Plant nutrients like indoles and quercetin from vegetables.

- Zinc – The best form may be zinc l-monomethionine (L-OptiZinc). Anyone who drinks alcohol must have this mineral, along with a B Complex vitamin.

- Milk Thistle – many herbs from many places in the world may help the liver. Probably the best studies are associated with this herb. It must be standardized. Dose matters and probably should be tailored.

❦

The FDA does not allow any specific nutrient health claims for nutrients. Therefore, consider this information as speculative and educational exploration. I cannot promise you that any nutrient or nutrient product will help you in any way.

End Notes

1. Belongia et al. Epidemiology and impact of coinfections acquired from Ixodes ticks. Vector Borne Zoonotic Dis. 2002 Winter; 2(4):265-73.

2. Rouqui P, Bodiga S and Raoult D. Eucarytic cells protect Borrelia burgdorferi from the action of penicillin and ceftriaxone but not from the action of doxycycline and erythromycin. Antimicrob Agents Chemother. 1996;40:1552-1554.

3. Steere AC, Malawista SE, Syndman DR. et al. Lyme arthritis: an epidemic of oigoarticular arthritis in children and adults in three Connecticut communities. Arthritis Rheum. 1977;Jan-Feb;20(1):7-17.

4. Scrimenti RJ. Erythema migrans. Arch Dermatol. 1970;102:104-105.

5. Steere AC. Lyme Disease. N Engl J Med. 1989;321:586-96.

6. Donta ST. Tetracycline therapy of chronic Lyme Disease. Clin Infect Dis. 1999;25:S52-56.

7. Donta ST. Treatment of chronic Lyme disease with macrolide antibiotics. In Program and abstracts of the VIIIth International Conference on Lyme Borreliosis. 1999 June 20-24; Munich, Germany. [Abstract p.193].

8. Bakken LL, Case KL, Callister SM, et al. Performance of 45 laboratories participating in a proficiency testing program for Lyme Disease serology. JAMA. 1992;268:891-895.

9. Fister RD, Weymouth LA, McLaughlin JC, et al.

Comparative evaluation of three products for the detection of Borrelia burgdorferi antibody in human serum. J Clin Microbil. 1989;37:2834-7.

10. Donta ST. Tetracycline therapy of chronic Lyme Disease. Clin Infect Dis. 1999;25:S52-56.

11. Donta ST. Treatment of chronic Lyme disease with macrolide antibiotics. In: Program and abstracts of the VIIIth International Conference on Lyme Borreliosis. 1999 June 20-24; Munich, Germany. [Abstract P193].

12. Belongia et al. Epidemiology and impact of coinfections acquired from Ixodes ticks. Vector Borne Zoonotic Dis. 2002 Winter;2(4):265-73.

13. Gutierrez Y. Blood apicomplexa: plasmodium, Babesia and entopolypoides. Ch 9. In: Diagnostic Pathology of Parasitic Infections with Clinical Correlations. Phila., PA. Lea Febiger. 1990; p.146.

14. Leeflang P, Oomen JMV, Zwart D, et al. The prevalence of Babesia antibodies in Nigerians. Int J Parasitol. 1976;6:156-161.

15. Osorno BM, Vega C, Ristic M, et al. Isolation of Babesia spp. from asymptomatic human beings. Vet. Parasitol. 1976;2:111-120.

16. DH, Mathiesen D, Glaser C, RS Lane, SR Telford III, JW Thomford, Mathieson D, Krause PJ, Phillip DF, and PA Conrad. Infection with a Babesia-like organism in north California. N Engl J Med. 1995;332:298-303.

17. Sonenshine DE. The biology of tick vectors of human disease. In: Tick-bourne Diseases of Humans. Edited by JL Goodman, DT Dennis, and Sonenshine DE.

Washington, DC. AMS Press. 2005;p.22-23.

18. Krause, PJ. Spielman, A, Telford, SR et al. Persistent parasitemia after acute Babesiosis. N. Engl. J. Med. 1998; 339:160.

19. Krause, PJ, Telford, SR, Spielman, A, et.al. Concurrent Lyme disease and Babesiosis. JAMA. 1996;275 (21):1657.

20. Stricker RB, Burrascano JJ, Harris NS, Horowitz R, Johnson L, Smith V, Phillips SE. Coinfection with Borrelia burgdorferi and Babesia microti: bad or worse? J Infect Dis. 2005;193:901-02.

21. Conrad PA, Kjemtrup AM, Carreno RA, Thomford J, Wainwright K, Eberhard M, Quick R, Telford III SR, Herwaldt BL. Description of Babesia duncani n.sp. (Apicomplexa: Babesiidae) from humans and its differentiation from other piroplasms. Int J Parasitol. 2006 May 4; [Epub ahead of print].

22. Hanafusa Y, Cho KO, Kanemaru T, Wada R, Sugimoto C, Onuma M. Pathogenesis of Babesia caballi infection in experimental horses. J Vet Med Sci. 1998 Oct;60(10):1127-32.

23. Final Diagnosis—Babesiosis. [cited 2006 Jul 3]. Available from: http://path.upmc.edu/cases/case332/dx. html.

24. Mylonakis, E. When to suspect and how to monitor babesiosis. American Family Physician. 2001;63:1969-74.

25. Persing DH, Herwaldt BL, Glaser C, Lane RS, Thomford JW, Mathiesen D, Krause PJ, Phillip DF,

Conrad PA. Infection with a Babesia-like organism in northern California. N Engl J Med.1995 Feb;2;332 (5):298-303.

26. Sherr VT. Babesiosis is an Underestimated, Unreported, but Serious Threat to the Nation's Health. 2006. In Press.

27. Andrew Schafley. Presentation at the 2005 American Association of Physicians and Surgeons.

28. Virginia T. Sherr. Human babesiosis – an unrecorded reality absence of formal registry undermines its detection, diagnosis and treatment, suggesting need for immediate mandatory reporting. Medical Hypotheses. 2004;63:609–615.

29. Virginia T. Sherr, MD. Babesiosis is an Underestimated, Unreported, but Serious Threat to the Nation's Health. In Press. 2006 Jun 30; [personal communication with email].

30. Virginia T. Sherr, MD. Babesiosis is an Underestimated, Unreported, but Serious Threat to the Nation's Health. In Press. 2006 Jun 30; [personal communication with email].

31. Moro MH, Zegarra-Moro OL, Bjornsson J, Hofmeister EK, Bruinsma E, Germer JJ, Persing DH. Increased arthritis severity in mice coinfected with Borrelia burgdorferi and Babesia microti. J Infec Dis. 2002 Aug 1;186(3):428-31. Epub 2002 Jul 5.

32. Zondervan. The Bible. Exodus. Ch 9;1-7 New International Version. 1984; Grand Rapids, Mich.

33. Marquardt WC, Demaree RS, Grieve R. Piroplasmea

and Piroplasmosis. In: Parasitology & Vector Biology, 2nd edition. San Diego, CA. Harcourt Press. 2000; p.221-224.

34. Marquardt WC, Demaree RS, Grieve R. Piroplasmea and Piroplasmosis. In: Parasitology & Vector Biology, 2nd edition. San Diego, CA. Harcourt Press. 2000; p.221-224.

35. Cunha BA, Barnett B, Sharma S, Talavera F, Sharma OP, Mylonakis E, Zevitz ME. Babesiosis. EMedicine. Accessed 2006 Jun 23.

36. Weiss LM. Babesiosis in humans: a treatment review. Expert Opinion Pharmacother. 202;3:1109.

37. Levine ND. Taxonomy of the pirolasms. Trans. Am. Microsc. Soc. 90:2-33.

38. Homer MJ, Aguiler-Delfin I, SR Telford III, PJ Krause and DH Persing. Babesiosis. Clinical Microbiology Reviews. 2000;13:451-469.

39. Telford SR III, Gorenflot A, Brasseur P and Spielman A. Babesial infections in hmans and wildlife. p.1-47. In: JP Kreier (ed.). Parasitic protozoa. 2nd ed. 1993;5. Academic Press. San Diego, Calif.

40. Lane RS, Moss RB, Hsu YP, Wei T, Mesirow ML, Kuo MM. Anti-arthropod saliva antibodies among residents of a community at high risk for Lyme disease in California. Am J Trop Med Hyg. 1999;61:850-9.

41. Bunnell JE, Price SD, Das A, Shields TM, Glass GE. Geographic information systems and spatial analysis of adult Ixodes scapularis (Acari: Ixodidae) in the MiddleAtlantic region of the USA. J Med Entomol.

2003;40(4):570-6.

42. Keirans JE, Hutcheson HJ, Durden LA, Klompen JS. Ixodes (Ixodes) scapularis (Acari:Ixodidae): redescription of all active stages, distribution, hosts, geographical variation, and medical and veterinary importance. J Med Entomol. 1996 May;33(3):297-318.

43. Wright SA, Lemenager DA, Tucker JR, Armijos MV, Yamamoto SA. An avian contribution to the presence of Ixodes pacificus (Acari: Ixodidae) and Borrelia burgdorferi on the sutter buttes of California. J Med Entomol. 2006 Mar;43(2):368-74.

44. Mitchell PD, Reed KD, Hofkes JM. Immunoserologic evidence of coinfection with Borrelia burgdorferi, Babesia microti, and human granulocytic Ehrlichia species in residents of Wisconsin and Minnesota. J Clin Microbiol. 1996 Mar;34(3):724-7.

45. Eskow ES, Krause PJ, Spielman A, Freeman K, Aslanzadeh J. Southern extension of the range of human babesiosis in the eastern United States. J Clin Microbiol. 1999 Jun;37(6):2051-2.

46. Hofmeister E, Kolbert C, Abdulkarim A, Magera J et al. Cosegregatin of a novel Bartonella species with Borrelia burgdorferi and Babesia microti in Peromyscus leucopus. J Infect Dis. 1998;177:409-416.

47. Setty S, Khalil Z, Schori P, Azar M, Ferrieri P. Babesiosis. Two atypical cases from Minnesota and a review. Am J Clin Pathol. 2003 Oct;120(4):554-9.

48. Virginia T. Sherr. Human babesiosis – an unrecorded reality absence of formal registry undermines its detec-

tion, diagnosis and treatment, suggesting need for immediate mandatory reporting. Medical Hypotheses. 2004;63:609-615.

49. Spielman A, Wilson ML, Levine JF, et al. Ecology of Ixodes dammini-borne human babesiosis and Lyme disease. Ann Rev Entomol. 1985;30:439-60.

50. Stafford KC, Massung RF, Magnarelli LA, Ijdo JW, Anderson JF. Infection with the agents of human granulocytic ehrlichiosis, Lyme disease, and babaesiosis in white-footed mice (Peromyscus leucopus) in Connecticut. J Clin Microbiol. 1999;37:2887-2.

51. Anderson JF, Mintz ED, Gadbaw JL, Magnerelli LA. Babesia microti, human babesiosis, and Borrelia burgdorferi in Connecticut. J. Clin Microbiol. 1991;29:2779-83.

52. VT Sherr. Unreported epidemic: failure to count cases of babesiosis. Bucks county courier times. 2000 July 6;6A:p.1.

53. Charles Ray Jones, MD. Personal Interview. 2005 Nov.

54. Hunfeld KP, Lambert A, Kampen H, Albert S, Epe C, Brade V, Tenter AM. Seroprevalence of Babesia infections in humans exposed to ticks in midwestern Germany. J Clin Microbiol. 2002 Jul;40(7):2431-6.

55. Piesman J, Mather TN, Dammin GJ,Telford SR 3rd, Lastavica CC, Spielman A. Seasonal variation of transmission risk of Lyme disease and human babesiosis. Am J Epidemiol. 1987 Dec;126(6):1187-9.

56. Belongia et al. Epidemiology and impact of coinfections acquired from Ixodes ticks. Vector Borne Zoonotic Dis.

2002 Winter;2(4):265-73.

57. Spielman A, Wilson ML, Levine JF, et al. Ecology of Ixodes dammini-borne human babesiosis and Lyme disease. Ann Rev Entomol. 1985;30:439-60.

58. Stafford KC, Massung RF, Magnarelli LA, Ijdo JW, Anderson JF. Infection with the agents of human granulocytic ehrlichIosis, Lyme disease, and babaesiosis in white-footed mice (Peromyscus leucopus) in Connecticut. J Clin Microbiol. 1999;37:2887-2.

59. Anderson JF, Mintz ED, Gadbaw JL, Magnerelli LA. Babesia microti, human babesiosis, and Borrelia burgdorferi in Connecticut. J Clin Microbiol. 1991;29:2779-83.

60. Mitchell PD, Reed KD, Hofkes JM. Immunoserologic evidence of coinfection with Borrelia burgdorferi, Babesia microti, and human granulocytic Ehrlichia species in residents of Wisconsin and Minnesota. J Clin Microbiol. 1996 Mar;34(3):724-7.

61. Benach JL, Coleman JL, Habicht GS, MacDonald A, Grunwaldt E, Giron JA. Serological evidence for simultaneous occurrences of Lyme disease and babesiosis. J Infect Dis. 1985 Sept;152(3):473-7.

62. Belongia et al. Epidemiology and impact of coinfections acquired from Ixodes ticks. Vector Borne Zoonotic Dis. 2002 Winter;2(4):265-73.

63. Adelson ME, Rao RV, Tilton RC, Cabets K, Eskow E, Fein L, Occi JL, Mordechai E. Prevalence of Borrelia burgdorferi, Bartonella spp., Babesia microti, and Anaplasma phagocytophila in Ixodes scapularis ticks

collected in Northern New Jersey. J Clin Microbiol. 2004 Jun;42(6):2799-801.

64.   Medical Diagnostic Laboratories L.L.C., 133 Gaither Dr., Suite C, Mt. Laurel, NJ 08054, USA. PCR analysis of Ixodes scapularis ticks collected in New Jersey identified infections with Borrelia burgdorferi (33.6%), Babesia microti (8.4%), Anaplasma phagocytophila (1.9%), and Bartonella spp. (34.5%). The I. Scapularis tick is a potential pathogen vector that can cause coinfection and contribute to the variety of clinical responses noted in some tick-borne disease patients. Cited in PubMed.

65.   Virginia T. Sherr. Human babesiosis – an unrecorded reality. Absence of formal registry undermines its detection, diagnosis and treatment, suggesting need for immediate mandatory reporting. Medical Hypotheses. 2004;63:609–615.

66.   Virginia T. Sherr. Babesiosis is an Underestimated, Unreported, but Serious Threat to the Nation's Health. 2004. In Press.

67.   Benach JL, Coleman JL, Habicht GS, MacDonald A, Grunwaldt E, Giron JA. Serological evidence for simultaneous occurrences of Lyme disease and babesiosis. J Infect Dis. 1985 Sept;152(3):473-7.

68.   Keirans JE, Hutcheson HJ, Durden LA, Klompen JS. Ixodes (Ixodes) scapularis (Acari:Ixodidae): redescription of all active stages, distribution, hosts, geographical variation, and medical and veterinary importance. J Med Entomol. 1996 May;33(3):297-318.

69. Mitchell PD, Reed KD, Hofkes JM. Immunoserologic evidence of coinfection with Borrelia burgdorferi, Babesia microti, and human granulocytic Ehrlichia species in residents of Wisconsin and Minnesota. J Clin Microbiol. 1996 Mar;34(3):724-7.

70. Marquardt WC, Demaree RS, Grieve R. Piroplasmea and Piroplasmosis. In: Parasitology & Vector Biology 2nd edition. San Diego, CA. Harcourt Press. 2000;p.221-224.

71. Persing DH, Herwaldt BL, Glaser C, Lane RS, Thomford JW, Mathiesen D, Krause PJ, Phillip DF, Conrad PA. Infection with a Babesia-like organism in northern California. N Engl J Med. 1995; 2;332:298-303.

72. Herwaldt RM, Kjemtrup AM, Conrad PA, Barnes RC, Wilson M, McCarthy MG, Sayers MH, Eberhard ML. Transfusion-transmitted babesiosis in Washington State: first reported case caused by WA1-type parasite. J. Infect. Dis. 1997;175:1259-1262.

73. Kjemtrup AM, Lee B, Fritz CL, Evans C, Chervenak M, Conrad PA. Investigation of transfusion transmission of a WA1-type babesial parasite to a premature infant in California. Transfusion. 2002;42:1482-7.

74. Quick RE, BL Herwaldt, JW Thomford, ME Garnett, ML Eberhard et al. Babesiosis in Washinton State: A New Species of Babesia? Annals of Internal Medicine. 119;284-290.

75. Thomford JW, Conrad PA, Telford SR II, Mathiesen D, et al. Cultivation and phylogenetic characterization of a

newly recognized human pathogenic protozoan. J Infectious Dis. 1994;169:1050-6.

76. Conrad PA, Kjemtrup AM, Carreno RA, Thomford J, Wainwright K, Eberhard M, Quick R, Telford III SR, Herwaldt BL. Description of Babesia duncani n.sp. (Apicomplexa: Babesiidae) from humans and its differentiation from other piroplasms. Int J Parasitol. 2006 May 4;[Epub ahead of print].

77. Conrad PA, Kjemtrup AM, Carreno RA, Thomford J, Wainwright K, Eberhard M, Quick R, Telford III SR, Herwaldt BL. Description of Babesia duncani n.sp. (Apicomplexa: Babesiidae) from humans and its differentiation from other piroplasms. Int J Parasitol. 2006 May 4;[Epub ahead of print].

78. Conrad PA, Kjemtrup AM, Carreno RA, Thomford J, Wainwright K, Eberhard M, Quick R, Telford III SR, Herwaldt BL. Description of Babesia duncani n.sp. (Apicomplexa: Babesiidae) from humans and its differentiation from other piroplasms. Int J Parasitol. 2006 May 4;[Epub ahead of print].

79. Persing DH, Herwaldt BL, Glaser C, Lane RS, Thomford JW, Mathiesen D, Krause PJ, Phillip DF, Conrad PA. Infection with a Babesia-like organism in northern California. N Engl J Med. 1995;2:332:298-303.

80. Herwaldt RM, Kjemtrup AM, Conrad PA, Barnes RC, Wilson M, McCarthy MG, Sayers MH, Eberhard ML. Transfusion-transmitted babesiosis in Washington State: first reported case caused by WA1-type parasite. J. Infect. Dis. 1997;175:1259-1262.

81. Kjemtrup AM, Lee B, Fritz CL, Evans C, Chervenak M, Conrad PA. Investigation of transfusion transmission of a WA1-type babesial parasite to a premature infant in California. Transfusion. 2002;42:1482-7.

82. Quick RE, BL Herwaldt, JW Thomford, ME Garnett, ML Eberhard et al. Babesiosis in Washinton State: A New Species of Babesia? Annals of Internal Medicine. 119;284-290.

83. JW Thomford, PA Conrad, SR Telford II, D Mathiesen, et al. Cultivation and phylogenetic characterization of a newly recognized human pathogenic protozoan. J Infectious Dis. 1994;169:1050-6.

84. Conrad PA, Kjemtrup AM, Carreno RA, Thomford J, Wainwright K, Eberhard M, Quick R, Telford III SR, Herwaldt BL. Description of Babesia duncani n.sp. (Apicomplexa: Babesiidae) from humans and its differentiation from other piroplasms. Int J Parasitol. 2006 May 4;[Epub ahead of print].

85. Herwaldt B, Persing DH, Precigout EA, Goff WL, Mathiesen DA, Taylor PW, Eberhard ML, Gorenflot AF. A fatal case of babesiosis in Missouri: identification of another piroplasm that infects humans. Ann Intern Med. 1997;126:172.

86. Steiner FE, Pinger RR, Vann CN, Abley MJ, Sullivan B, Grindle N, Clay K, Fuqua C. Detection of Anaplasma phagocytophilum and Babesia odocoilei DNA in Ixodes scapularis (Acari: Ixodidae) collected in Indiana. J Med Entomol. 2006;43:437-42.

87. Armstrong PM, Katavolos P, Caporale DA, Smith RP,

Spielman A, Telford SR III. Diversity of Babesia infecting deer ticks (Ixodes dammini). Am J Trop Med Hyg. 1998;58:739-42.

88. Gorenflot A, Moubri K, Precigout G, Carcy B, Schetters TP. Human babesiosis. Ann. The severity Trop. Med. Parisitol. 1998;92:489-501.

89. Hunfeld KP, Brade V. Zoonotic Babesia: Possibly emerging pathogens to be considered for tick-infested humans in central Europe. Int. J. Med. Microbiol. 2004;S37:93-103.

90. Faulde M, Hoffmann G. Vorkommen und Verhutung vertorassoziierter Erkrankungen des Menschen in Deutschland unter Berucksichtigung zoonotischer Aspekte. Bundesgesundheitsbl. – Gesundheitsforsch. – Gesundheitsschutz. 2001;44:116-136.

91. Herwaldt BL, Caccio S, Gherlinzoni F, Aspock H, Slemenda SB, Piccaluga P, Martinelli G, Edelhofer R, Hollenstein U, Poletti G, Pampiglione S, Loschenberger K, Tura S, and NJ Pieniazek. Molecular characterization of a non-Babesia divergens organism causing zoonotic babesiosis in Europe. Emerging Infectious Diseases. 2000;9;942-948.

92. Mathis A, Hilpertshauser H, Deplazes P. [Piroplasms of ruminants in Switzerland and zoonotic significance of Babesia]. Schweiz Arch Tierheilkd. 2006;148:151-9.

93. Herwaldt BL, Caccio S, Gherlinzoni F, Aspock H, Slemenda SB, Piccaluga P, Martinelli G, Edelhofer R, Hollenstein U, Poletti G, Pampiglione S, Loschenberger K, Tura S, Pieniazek NJ. Molecular characterization of a

non-Babesia divergens organism causing zoonotic babesiosis in Europe. Emerg Infect Dis. 2003;9:942-8.

94. Jacquemin L, Bazin C, Lamy C, Chubilleau C, Barale T, Daoudal P, Duhamel C. Babesiose (ou piroplasmose) humaine: a propos de trios observations recentes en France. Maghreb Informations Medicales. 1980;2:31-38.

95. Calvo de Mora A, Garcia Castellano JM, Herrera C and Jimenez-Alonso J. Babesiosis humana: aportacion de un caso de evolucion fatal. Medicina Clinia. 1985;85:515-516.

96. Skrabalo Z, Deanovic Z. Piroplasmosis in man. Documenta de Medicina Geographica et Tropica. 1957;9:11-16.

97. Thomford JW, Conrad PA, Telford SR, Mathiesen M, Bowman BH, Spielman A, Eberhard ML, Herwaldt BL, Quick RE, and DH Persing. Cultivation and Phylogenetic Characterization of a Newly Recognized Human Pathogenic Protozoan. J Infect Dis. 1994;169:1050-1056.

98. Setty S, Khalil Z, Schori P, Azar M, Ferrieri P. Babesiosis. Two atypical cases from Minnesota and a review. Am J Clin Pathol. 2003;120:554-9.

99. Herwaldt BL, Caccio S, Gherlinzoni F, Aspock H, Slemenda SB, Piccaluga P Martinelli G, Edelhofer R, Hollenstein U, Poletti G, Pampiglione S, Loschenberger K, Tura S, and NJ Pieniazek. Molecular characterization of a non-Babesia divergens organism causing zoonotic babesiosis in Europe. Emerging Infectious Diseases. 2000;9:942-948.

100. Mathis A, Hilpertshauser H, Deplazes P. [Piroplasms of ruminants in Switzerland and zoonotic significance of Babesia]. Schweiz Arch Tierheilkd. 2006;148:151-9.

101. Ohrt C, Purnomo, Sutamihardja MA, Tang D, Kain KC. Impact of microscopy error on estimates of protective efficacy in malaria-prevention trials. J Infect Dis. 2002 Aug;15;186(4):540-6. [Epub. 2002 Aug 2].

102. Cabezos J, Bada JL. The diagnosis of malaria by the thick film and the QBC: a comparative study of both technics. Med Clin (Barc). 1993 Jun 12;101(3):91-4.

103. Hanscheid T, Melo-Cristino J, Grobusch MP, Pinto BG. Avoiding misdiagnosis of imported malaria: screening of emergency department samples with thrombocytopenia detects clinically unsuspected cases. J Travel Med. 2003 May-Jun;10(3):155-9.

104. Collier JA, Longmore JM. The reliability of the microscopic diagnosis of malaria in the field and in the laboratory. Ann Trop Med Parasitol. 1983 Apr;77(2):113-7.

105. Ohnishi K, Murata M. Malaria–eight years of experience in a Tokyo metropolitan hospital. Intern Med. 1996 Feb;35(2):111-4.

106. Kachur SP, Reller ME, Barber AM, Barat LM, Koumans EH, Parise ME, Roberts J, Ruebush TK 2nd, Zucker JR. Malaria surveillance–United States, 1994. MMWR. CDC Surveill. Summ. 1997;Oct 17;46(5):1-18.

107. Moore TA, Tomayko JF Jr, Wierman AM, Rensimer ER, White AC Jr. Imported malaria in the 1990s. A report of 59 cases from Houston, Tex. 30. Arch Fam Med. 1994 Feb;3(2):130-6.

108. Bruckner DA, Garcia LS, Shimizu RY, Goldstein EJ, Murray PM, Lazar GS. Babesiosis: problems in diagnosis using autoanalyzers, Am J Clin Pathol. 1985 Apr;83(4):520-1.

109. MacDonald, PhD. Repeated personal communication, June;2006.

110. Burrascano, Joseph J. Advanced topics in Lyme Disease: Diagnostic Hints and Treatment Guidelines for Lyme and other Tick borne Illnesses. Fifteenth Edition, September 2005. Available from: http://www.personal-consult.com/articles/moldandbiotoxins/advanced burrascano.html.

111. Wright IG, Goodger BV, Clark IA. Immuno-pathophysiology of Babesia bovis and Plasmodium falciparum infections. Babesia. Malaria Treatment. Parasitol Today. 1988 Aug;4(8):214-8.

112. Krause PJ. Babesiosis diagnosis and treatment. Vector Borne Zoonotic Dis. 2003;3:45-51.

113. Atovaquone. Drug Facts and Comparisons 2006. Wolters Kluwer Health. St. Louis, Missouri; p.1915.

114. Babesiosis". Family Practice Notebook.com. Available from: http://fnotebook.com/ID219.htm. Accessed June 30, 2006.

115. Rencricca NJ, Cleman RM, Altschule MD, et al. Quantification of hyperbaric oxygen-induced toxicity utilizing a malarial system. Aviat space environ med. 1981;52:85-87.

116. Parapini S, Basilico N, Mondani M, et al. Evidence that haem iron in the malaria parasite is not needed for the

antimalarial effects of artemisinin. FEBS Lett. 2004;575:p.91-94.

117. Krause PJ, Lepore T, Sikand VK, Gadbaw J Jr, Burke G, Telford SR III, Brassard P, Pearl D, Azlanzadeh J, Christianson D, McGrath D, Spielman A. Atovaquone and azithromycin for the treatment of babesiosis. New England Journal of Medicine. 2000;343:1454-8.

118. Krause PJ. Babesiosis. Medical Clinics of North America. March 2002;Vol. 86. [cited 2006 Aug]. Available from: http://home.mdconsult.com.

119. CF Lacy, LL Armstrong, MP Goldman, LL Lance. Drug Information Handbook. 14th edition. Hudson, Ohio: Lexi-Comp; 2006. p. 175-176.

120. CF Lacy, LL Armstrong, MP Goldman, LL Lance. Drug Information Handbook. 14th edition. Hudson, Ohio: Lexi-Comp; 2006. p. 175-176.

121. The use of artemisinin and its derivatives as anti-malarial drugs. WHO/MAL/98.1086. Malaria Unit, Division of Control of Tropical Diseases, WHO, Geneva. 1998.

122. Wilairatana P, Looaresuwan S. The clinical use of artemisinin and its derivatives in the treatment of malaria. In Artemesia, Wright, CW, Ed. Taylor & Francis, London. 2002;p.298-299.

123. Singh NP, Lai HC. Synergistic cytotoxicity of artemisinin and sodium butyrate on human cancer cells. Anticancer Res. 2005;25(6B):4325-31.

124. Berger TG, Dieckmann D, Efferth T, Schultz ES, Funk JO, Baur A, Schuler G. Artesunate in the treatment of metastatic uveal melanoma–first experiences. Oncol

Rep. 2005;14:1599-603.

125. Efferth T, Dunstan H, Sauerbrey A, Miyachi H, Chitambar CR. The anti-malarial artesunate is also active against cancer. Int J Oncol. 2001 Apr;18(4):767-73.

126. J.F.S. Ferreira and J. Janick. Distribution of artemisinin in Artemisia annua. p.579-584. In: J. Janick (ed.), Progress in new crops. 1996;ASHS Press, Arlington, VA.

127. Klayman D. Qinghaosu (Artemisinin): Antimalarial Drug from China. Science, 1985, May 31;238:p.1049.

128. Eds. M. Willcox, G. Bodeker, G. Bourdy et al. Artemesia annua as a traditional herbal antimalarial. In: Traditional Medicinal Plants and Malaria. Eds. M. Willcox, G. Bodeker, P. Rasoanaivo. New York,CRC Press;2004;p.46.

129. The World Health Organization. Roll Back Malaria Infosheet. Facts on ACTs (Artemisinin-based Combination Therapies), An Update on Recent Progress in Policy and Access to Treatment. Available from: http://www.rbm.who.int/cmc_upload/0/000/015/ 364/RB-MInfosheet_9.htm. Accessed 2006 Aug 10.

130. Hasslberger, S. Sweet Wormwood Heals Malaria. [monograph on the Internet]. Available from: http://www.newmediaexplorer.org/sepp/2004/07/17/sweet_w ormwood_heals_malaria.htm. Accessed 2006 Aug 1.

131. The World Health Organization. Roll Back Malaria Infosheet. Facts on ACTs (Artemisinin-based Combination Therapies), An Update on Recent Progress in Policy and Access to Treatment. Available from: http://www.rbm.who.int/cmc_upload/0/000/015/

364/RB-MInfosheet_9.htm. Accessed 2006 Aug 10.

132. Hasslberger, S. Sweet Wormwood Heals Malaria. Available from: http://www.newmediaexplorer.org/ sepp/2004/07/17/sweet_wormwood_heals_malaria.htm. Accessed 2006, Aug 1.

133. The World Health Organization. Roll Back Malaria Infosheet. Facts on ACTs (Artemisinin-based Combination Therapies), An Update on Recent Progress in Policy and Access to Treatment. Available from: http://www.rbm.who.int/cmc_upload/0/000/ 015/364/RB-MInfosheet_9.htm. Accessed 2006 Aug 10.

134. McNeil DG Jr. Plant shortage leaves campaigns against malaria at risk. New York Times. 2004 Nov 14. [cited 2006 Jul]. Available from: http://www.nytimes.com/ 2004/11/14/international/asia/14malaria.html?ex=11344 50000&en=7ce7c3af52873986&ei=5070.

135. WHO and UNICEF. Global Financing, Commodities and Service Delivery. World Malaria Report 2005. [cited 2006 Jul]. Available from: http://rbm.who.int/wmr2005/ html/3-1.htm.

136. Ro DK, Paradise EM, Ouellet M, Fisher KJ, Newman KL, Ndungu JM, Ho KA, Eachus RA, Ham TS, Kirby J, Chang MC, Withers ST, Shiba Y, Sarpong R, Keasling JD. Production of the antimalarial drug precursor artemisinic acid in engineered yeast. Nature. 2006 Apr 13;440(7086):852-3 [and] 940-3. Accessed 2006 Aug 12.

137. McNeil DG Jr. Plant shortage leaves campaigns against malaria at risk. New York Times. 2004 Nov 14. [cited 2006 Jul]. Available from: http://www. nytimes.com/

2004/11/14/international/asia/14malaria.html?ex=11344 50000&en=7ce7c3af52873986&ei=5070.

138. Purcell, K. Gates Foundation Invests $42.6 Million in Malaria Drug Research. American Botanical Council. [homepage on the Internet]. HerbalGram. 2006;69:24-252. Available from: http://www.herbalgram.org/ herbalgram/articleview.asp?a=2919. Accessed 2006 Aug 10.

139. Medical News Today. [Monograph on the Internet]. Available from: http://www.medicalnewstoday.com/medical-news.php?newsid=3518. Accessed 2006 Aug 13.

140. Purcell, Katherine. Gates Foundation Invests $42.6 Million in Malaria Drug Research. From: HerbalGram. American Botanical Council. 2006;69:24-252. Available from: http://www.herbalgram.org/herbalgram/article-view.asp?a=2919. Accessed 2006 Aug 13.

141. Zhang Q, Zhang Y. Lyme disease and modern Chinese medicine. Sino-Med Reseach Institute, New York, NY. 2006;p.34-35.

142. Nandakumar DN, Nagaraj VA, Vathsala PG, Rangarajan P, Padmanaban G. Curcumin-artemisinin combination therapy for malaria. Antimicrob Agents Chemother. 2006 May;50(5):1859-60.

143. China Cooperative Research Group on Qinghaosu and its Derivatives as Antimalarials. J. Trad. Chin. Med. 1982;217.

144. Robert Jay Rowen, Artemisinin: From Malaria to Cancer Treatment. Townsend Letter for Doctors & Patients, 2002 Dec.

145. Augustijns P, D'Hulst A, Van Daele J, Kinget R.

Transport of artemisinin and sodium artesunate in Caco-2 intestinal epithelial cells. J Pharm Sci. 1996 Jun;85(6):577-9.

146. Svensson US, Sandstrom R, Carlborg O, Lennernas H, Ashton M. High in situ rat intestinal permeability of artemisinin unaffected by multiple dosing and with no evidence of P-glycoprotein involvement. Drug Metab Dispos. 1999;27:227-32.

147. de Vries PJ, Dien TK. Clinical pharmacology and therapeutic potential of artemisinin and its derivatives in the treatment of malaria. Drugs. 1996;52:818-36.

148. Panossian LA, Garga NI, Pelletier D. Toxic brainstem encephalopathy after artemisinin treatment for breast cancer. Ann. Neurol 2005;56;812-813.

149. Gordi T, Xie R, Huong NV, Huong DX, Karlsson MO, Ashton M. A semiphysiological pharmacokinetic model for artemisinin in healthy subjects incorporating autoinduction of metabolism and saturable first-pass hepatic extraction. Br J Clin Pharmacol. 2005 Feb;59(2):189-98.

150. Van Agtmael MA, Eggelte TA and CJ van Boxtel. Artmisinin drugs in the treatment of malaria: from medicinal herb to registered medication. Trends Pharmacol. Sci. 1999;20:199-205.

151. Wong JW, Yuen KH, Nagappan S, Shahul WS, Ho SS, Gan EK, Toh WT. Therapeutic equivalence of a low dose artemisinin formulation in falciparum malaria patients. J Pharm Pharmacol. 2003 Feb;55(2):193-8.

152. Phillips-Howard P. Regulation of the quality and use of artemisinin and its derivatives. In: Artemisia. Wright

CW. Ed. 2002: Taylor and Francis, London.

153. Van Agtmael MA, Eggelte TA and CJ van Boxtel. Artmisinin drugs in the treatment of malaria: from medicinal herb to registered medication. Trends Pharmacol. Sci. 1999;20:199-205.

154. Wong JW, Yuen KH, Nagappan S, Shahul WS, Ho SS, Gan EK, Toh WT. Therapeutic equivalence of a low dose artemisinin formulation in falciparum malaria patients. J Pharm Pharmacol. 2003;55:193-8.

155. Phillips-Howard P. Regulation of the quality and use of artemisinin and its derivatives. In: Artemisia. Wright CW. Ed. 2002: Taylor and Francis, London.

156. Willcox M, Bodeker G, Bourdy G et al. Artemesia annua as a traditional herbal antimalarial. In: Traditional Medicinal Plants and Malaria. Eds. M. Willcox, G. Bodeker, P. Rasoanaivo. New York: CRC Press, 2004;p.48-50.

157. Na-Bangchang K, Krudsood S, Silachamroon U, Molunto P, Tasanor O, Chalermrut K, Tangpukdee N, Matangkasombut O, Kano S, Looareesuwan S. The pharmacokinetics of oral dihydroartemisinin and artesunate in healthy Thai volunteers. Southeast Asian J Trop Med Public Health. 2004 Sept;35(3):575-82.

158. Looaresuwan S, Wilairatana P, Vanijanonta S, et al. Treatment of acute, uncomplicated, falciparum malaria with oral dihydroartemisinin. Ann Trop Med Parasitol. 1996;90:21-28.

159. Van Agtmael MA, Gupta V, van der Wosten, et al. Grapefruit juice increases the bioavailability of

artemether. Eur. J. Clin. Pharmacol. 1999;55:405-410.

160. Suputtamongkol Y, Newton PN, Angus B, Teja-Isavadharm P, Keeratithakul D, Rasameesoraj M, Pukrittayakamee S, White NJ. A comparison of oral artesunate and artemether antimalarial bioactivities in acute falciparum malaria. Br J Clin Pharmacol. 2001 Dec;52(6):655-61.

161. de Vries PJ, Dien TK. Clinical pharmacology and therapeutic potential of artemisinin and its derivatives in the treatment of malaria. Drugs. 1996 Dec;52(6):818-36.

162. Suputtamongkol Y, Newton PN, Angus B, Teja-Isavadharm P, Keeratithakul D, Rasameesoraj M, Pukrittayakamee S, White NJ. A comparison of oral artesunate and artemether antimalarial bioactivities in acute falciparum malaria. Br J Clin Pharmacol. 2001 Dec;52(6):655-61.

163. Wilairatana P, Looaresuwan S. The clinical use of artemisinin and its derivatives in the treatment of malaria. In Artemesia, Wright, CW, Ed. Taylor & Francis, London. 2002;p.291-306.

164. Nealon C, Dzeing A, Muller-Romer U, Planche T, Sinou V, Kombila M, Kremsner PG, Parzy D, Krishna S. Intramuscular bioavailability and clinical efficacy of artesunate in gabonese children with severe malaria. Antimicrob Agents Chemother. 2002 Dec;46(12):3933-9.

165. Olliaro PL, Nair NK, Sathasivam K, Mansor SM, Navaratnam V. Pharmacokinetics of artesunate after single oral administration to rats. BMC Pharmacol. 2001;1:12. [Epub. 2001 Dec 20].

166. Batty KT, Davis TM, Thu LT et al. Selective high-performance liquid chromatographic determination of artesunate and alpha- and beta-dihydroartemisinin in patients with falciparum malaria. J Chromatogr B Biomed Appl. 1996;677:345-350.

167. Batty KT, Thu LT, Davis TM, Ilett KF, Mai TX, Hung NC, Tien NP, Powell SM, Thien HV, Binh TQ, Kim NV. A pharmacokinetic and pharmacodynamic study of intravenous vs oral artesunate in uncomplicated falciparum malaria. Br J Clin Pharmacol. 1998;45:123-9.

168. Batty KT, Iletr KE, Powell SM, Martin J, Davis TM. Relative bioavailability of artesunate and dihydroartemisinin: investigations in the isolated perfused rat liver and in healthy Caucasian volunteers. Am J Trop Med Hyg. 2002;66:130-6.

169. Hayes RK. From artemisinin to new artemisinin antimalarials: bio-synthesis, extraction, old and new derivatives, stereochemistry and medicinal chemistry requirements. Current Topics in Medicinal Chemistry. 2006;6:509-537.

170. Sabarinath SN, Asthana OP, Puri SK, Srivastava K, Madhusudanan KP, Gupta RC. Clinical pharmacokinetics of the diastereomers of arteether in healthy volunteers. Clin Pharmacokinet. 2005;44(11):1191-203.

171. Sabarinath S, Madhusudanan KP, Gupta RC. Pharmacokinetics of the diastereomers of arteether, a potent antimalarial drug, in rats. Biopharm Drug Dispos. 2005 Sept;26(6):211-23.

172. Zhang Q, Zhang Y. Lyme disease and modern Chinese

medicine. Sino-Med Reseach Institute, New York, NY: 2006;p.76-82.

173. Zhang Q, Zhang Y. Lyme disease and modern Chinese medicine. Sino-Med Reseach Institute, New York, NY: 2006;p.1-5.

174. Benakis A, Binh TQ, Keundjian A, Scheiwe MW. Pharmacokinetics/Pharmacodynamics findings after repeated administration of ARTESUNATE thermostable suppositories (RECTOCAPS) in Vietnamese patients with uncomplicated malaria. Eur J Drug Metab Pharmacokinet. 2006 Jan-Mar;31(1):41-5.

175. Lin AJ, Ager AL Jr, Klayman DL. Antimalarial activity of dihydroartemisinin derivatives by transdermal application. Am J Trop Med Hyg. 1994 Jun;50(6):777-83.

176. Klayman DL, Ager AL Jr, Fleckenstein L, Lin AJ. Transdermal artelinic acid: an effective treatment for Plasmodium berghei-infected mice. Am J Trop Med Hyg. 1991 Nov;45(5):602-7.

177. Zhao KC, Xuan WY, Zhao Y, Song ZY. The pharmacokinetics of a transdermal preparation of artesunate in mice and rabbits.Yao Xue Xue Bao. 1989;24(11):813-6.

178. Thriemer K, Wernsdorfer G, Rojanawatsirivet C, Kollaritsch H, Sirichainsinthop J, Wernsdorfer WH. In vitro activity of artemisinin alone and in combination with retinol against Plasmodium falciparum. Wien Klin Wochenschr. 2005;117 Suppl. 4:45-8.

179. LaValle JA, Krinsky DL, Hawkin EB, Pelton R and A Ashbrook Willlis. Natural Therapeutics Pocket Guide 2000-2001. Hudson, OH;Lexi-Comp. 518,531.

180. Michael Lam, Artemisinin (Wormwood) – From Malaria To Cancer. [Monograph on the Internet]. [cited 2006 Aug]. Available from: http://www.drlam.com/ A3R_brief_in_doc_format/Artemisinin.cfm.

181. Galal AM, Ross SA, ElSohly MA, ElSohly HN, El-Feraly FS, Ahmed MS, McPhail AT. Deoxyartemisinin derivatives from photooxygenation of anhydrodeoxydi-hydroartemisinin and their cytotoxic evaluation. J Nat Prod. 2002;65:184-8.

182. Lee CH, Hong H, Shin J, Jung M, Shin I, Yoon J, Lee W. NMR studies on novel antitumor drug candidates, deoxoartemisinin and carboxypropyldeoxoartemisinin. Biochem Biophys Res Commun. 2000;274:359-69.

183. Singh NP, Lai HC. Synergistic cytotoxicity of artemisinin and sodium butyrate on human cancer cells. Anticancer Res. 2005 Nov-Dec;25(6B):4325-31.

184. Butler AR, Gilbert BC, Hulme P, Irvine LR, Rendon L, Whitwood AC. EPR evidence for the involvement of free radicals in the iron-catalysed decomposition of quinghaosu (artemisinin) and some derivatives; anti-malarial action of some polycyclic endoperoxides. Free Radic Res. 1998 May;28(5):471-6.

185. Sun WC, Han JX, Yang WY, Deng DA, Yue XF. Antitumor activities of 4 derivatives of artemisic acid and artemisinin B in vitro. Zhongguo Yao Li Xue Bao. 1992;13:541-3. Erratum in: Chung Kuo Yao Li Hsueh Pao 1993;14:192. [Article in Chinese].

186. Lee J, Zhou HJ, Wu XH. Dihydroartemisinin downregu-lates vascular endothelial growth factor expression and

induces apoptosis in chronic myeloid leukemia K562 cells. Cancer Chemother Pharmacol. 2006 Jan;57(2):213-20. [Epub 2005 Aug 2].

187. Berger TG, Dieckmann D, Efferth T, Schultz ES, Funk JO, Baur A, Schuler G. Artesunate in the treatment of metastatic uveal melanoma–first experiences. Oncol Rep. 2005 Dec;14(6):1599-603.

188. Efferth T, Olbrich A, Bauer R. mRNA expression profiles for the response of human tumor cell lines to the antimalarial drugs artesunate, arteether, and artemether. Biochem Pharmacol. 2002;64:617-23.

189. Singh NP, Lai HC. Synergistic cytotoxicity of artemisinin and sodium butyrate on human cancer cells. Anticancer Res. 2005;25:4325-31.

190. Lai H, Singh NP. Oral artemisinin prevents and delays the development of 7,12-dimethylbenz[a]anthracene (DMBA)-induced breast cancer in the rat. Cancer Lett. 2006;231:43-8.

191. Singh NP, Lai H. Selective toxicity of dihydroartemisinin and holotransferrin toward human breast cancer cells. Life Sci. 2001;70(1):49-56.

192. Posner GH, McRiner AJ, Paik IH, Sur S, Borstnik K, Xie S, Shapiro TA, Alagbala A, Foster B. Anticancer and antimalarial efficacy and safety of artemisinin-derived trioxane dimers in rodents. J Med Chem. 2004;47:1299-301.

193. Kim SJ, Kim MS, Lee JW, Lee CH, Yoo H, Shin SH, Park MJ, Lee SH. Dihydroartemisinin enhances radiosensitivity of human glioma cells in vitro. J Cancer

Res Clin Oncol. 2006;132:129-35. [Epub 2005 Nov 5].

194. Efferth T. Molecular pharmacology and pharmacogenomics of artemisinin and its derivatives in cancer cells. Curr Drug Targets. 2006; 7:407-21.

195. Anfosso L, Efferth T, Albini A, Pfeffer U. Microarray expression profiles of angiogenesis-related genes predict tumor cell response to artemisinins. Pharmacogenomics J. 2006;6:269-78. [Epub 2006 Jan 24].

196. Paik IH, Xie S, Shapiro TA, Labonte T, Narducci Sarjeant AA, Baege AC, Posner GH. Second generation, orally active, antimalarial, artemisinin-derived trioxane dimers with high stability, efficacy, and anticancer activity. J Med Chem. 2006;49:2731-4.

197. Galal AM, Ross SA, ElSohly MA, ElSohly HN, El-Feraly FS, Ahmed MS, McPhail AT. Deoxyartemisinin derivatives from photooxygenation of anhydrodeoxydihydroartemisinin and their cytotoxic evaluation. J Nat Prod. 2002;65:184-8.

198. Lee CH, Hong H, Shin J, Jung M, Shin I, Yoon J, Lee W. NMR studies on novel antitumor drug candidates, deoxoartemisinin and carboxypropyldeoxoartemisinin. Biochem Biophys Res Commun. 2000;274:359-69.

199. Disbrow GL, Baege AC, Kierpiec KA, Yuan H, Centeno JA, Thibodeaux CA, Hartmann D, Schlegel R. Dihydroartemisinin is cytotoxic to papillomavirus-expressing epithelial cells in vitro and in vivo. Cancer Res. 2005;65:10854-61.

200. Chen HH, Zhou HJ, Fang X. Inhibition of human cancer cell line growth and human umbilical vein endothelial

cell angiogenesis by artemisinin derivatives in vitro. [cervical cancer]. Pharmacol Res. 2003;48:231-6.

201. Liu Y, Wong VK, Ko BC, Wong MK, Che CM. Synthesis and cytotoxicity studies of artemisinin derivatives containing lipophilic alkyl carbon chains. Org Lett. 2005;7:1561-4.

202. Sun WC, Han JX, Yang WY, Deng DA, Yue XF. Antitumor activities of 4 derivatives of artemisic acid and artemisinin B in vitro. Zhongguo Yao Li Xue Bao. 1992;13:541-3. Erratum in: Chung Kuo Yao Li Hsueh Pao 1993;14:192. [Article in Chinese].

203. Dell'Eva R, Pfeffer U, Vene R, Anfosso L, Forlani A, Albini A, Ef-ferth T. Inhibition of angiogenesis in vivo and growth of Kaposi's sarcoma xenograft tumors by the anti-malarial artesunate. Bio-chem Pharmacol. 2004;68:2359-66.

204. Efferth T, Benakis A, Romero MR, Tomicic M, Rauh R, Steinbach D, Hafer R, Stamminger T, Oesch F, Kaina B, Marschall M. Enhancement of cytotoxicity of artemisinins toward cancer cells by ferrous iron. Free Radic Biol Med. 2004 Oct 1;37(7):998-1009.

205. Singh NP, Lai HC. Artemisinin induces apoptosis in human cancer cells. Anticancer Res. 2004;24:2277-80.

206. Moore JC, Lai H, Li JR, Ren RL, McDougall JA, Singh NP, Chou CK. Oral administration of dihydroartemisinin and ferrous sulfate retarded implanted fibrosarcoma growth in the rat. Cancer Lett. 1995 Nov;98(1):83-7.

207. Yamachika E, Habte T, Oda D. Artemisinin: an alternative treatment for oral squamous cell carcinoma.

Anticancer Res. 2004;24:2153-60.

208. Chen HH, Zhou HJ, Wu GD, Lou XE. Inhibitory effects of artesunate on angiogenesis and on expressions of vascular endothelial growth factor and VEGF receptor KDR/flk-1. Pharmacology. 2004;71:1-9.

209. Chen HH, Zhou HJ, Fang X. Inhibition of human cancer cell line growth and human umbilical vein endothelial cell angiogenesis by artemisinin derivatives in vitro. Pharmacol Res. 2003;48:231-6.

210. Sadava D, Phillips T, Lin C, Kane SE. Transferrin overcomes drug resistance to artemisinin in human small-cell lung carcinoma cells. Cancer Lett. 2002;179:151-6.

211. Sun WC, Han JX, Yang WY, Deng DA, Yue XF. Antitumor activi-ties of 4 derivatives of artemisic acid and artemisinin B in vitro. Zhongguo Yao Li Xue Bao. 1992 Nov;13(6):541-3. Erratum in: Chung Kuo Yao Li Hsueh Pao 1993;14:192. [Article in Chinese].

212. Sun WC, Han JX, Yang WY, Deng DA, Yue XF. Antitumor activities of 4 derivatives of artemisic acid and artemisinin B in vitro. Zhongguo Yao Li Xue Bao. 1992;13:541-3. Erratum in: Chung Kuo Yao Li Hsueh Pao 1993;14:192. [Article in Chinese].

213. Lai H., Narendra S. Cancer Letters. 1995;91:41-46.

214. May WS. J Membr. Biol. 1985;88:205-215.

215. Singh NP, Lai H. Life Sci. 2001;70:49-56.

216. Kakkilaya, BS. The Malaria Site. Malaria Risk in Africa. Available from: http://www.malariasite.com/malaria/artemisinin.htm. Accessed August 13, 2006.

217. Hasslberger, S. Sweet Wormwood Heals Malaria. Available from: http://www.newmediaexplorer.org/sepp/2004/07/17/sweet_wormwood_heals_malaria.htm. Accessed 17, 2006.

218. The World Health Organization. Roll Back Malaria Infosheet. [monograph on the Internet]. Facts on ACTs (Artemisinin-based Combination Therapies), An Update on Recent Progress in Policy and Access to Treatment. Available from: http://www. rbm.who.int/cmc_upload/0/000/015/364/RBMInfosheet_9.htm. Accessed August 10, 2006.

219. Olsen A, Nawiri J, Magnussen P, Krarup H, Friis H. Failure of twice-weekly iron supplementation to increase blood haemoglobin and serum ferritin concentrations: results of a randomized controlled trial. Ann Trop Med Parasitol. 2006 Apr;100(3):251-63.

220. Schaller JA, MD. Personal regular monthly communications. 1996-2000.

221. Messori L, Gabbiani C, Casini A, Siragusa M, Vincieri FF, Bilia AR. The reaction of artemisinins with hemoglobin: a unified picture. Bioorg Med Chem. 2006 May 1;14(9):2972-7. [Epub 2006 Jan 10].

222. Selmeczi K, Robert A, Claparols C, Meunier B. Alkylation of human hemoglobin by the antimalarial drug artemisinin. FEBS Lett. 2004 Jan 2;(1-3):245-48,556.

223. Kim SJ, Kim MS, Lee JW, Lee CH, Yoo H, Shin SH, Park MJ, Lee SH. Dihydroartemisinin enhances radiosensitivity of human glioma cells in vitro. J Cancer

Res Clin Oncol. 2006 Feb;132(2):129-35. [Epub 2005 Nov 5].

224. Murray MT. Encyclopedia of Nutritional Supplements. Prima; Rocklin, CA 1996;p.208-13.

225. Dondorp AM, Omodeo-Sale F, Chotivanich K, Taramelli D, White NJ. Oxidative stress and rheology in severe malaria. Redox Rep. 2003;8:292-4.

226. Ames JR, Ryan MD, Klayman DL. Charge transfer and oxy radicals in antimalarial action. J. Free Rad Biol. Med. 1985;1:353-61.

227. Krungkrai SR, Yuthavong. The antimalarial action of Plasmodium falciparum of qinghaosu and artesunate in combination with agents which modulate oxidant stress. Trans. R Soc. Trop. Med Hyg 1987;81:710-4.

228. Levander OA, Ager AL, Morris VC. Qinghaosu, dietary vitamin E, selenium and cod liver oil: effect on susceptibility of mice to the malarial parasite Plasmodium yoelii. Am. J. Clin. Nutr. 1989;5:346-52.

229. Kim SJ, Kim MS, Lee JW, Lee CH, Yoo H, Shin SH, Park MJ, Lee SH. Dihydroartemisinin enhances radiosensitivity of human glioma cells in vitro. J Cancer Res Clin Oncol. 2006 Feb;132(2):129-35. [Epub 2005 Nov 5].

230. Spapen H, Zhang H, Demanet C, et al. Does N-acetyl-L-cysteine influence cytokine response during early human septic shock. Chest. 1998;113:1616-24.

231. Dondorp AM, Omodeo-Sale F, Chotivanich K, Taramelli D, White NJ. Oxidative stress and rheology in severe malaria. Redox Rep. 2003;8(5):292-4.

232. Watt G, Jongsakul K, Ruangvirayuth R. A pilot study of N-acetylcysteine as adjunctive therapy for severe malaria. QJM. 2002 May;95(5):285-90.

233. Treeprasertsuk S, Krudsood S, Tosukhowong T, Maek-A-Nantawat W, Vannaphan S, Saengnetswang T, Looareesuwan S, Kuhn WF, Brittenham G, Carroll J. N-acetylcysteine in severe falciparum malaria in Thailand. Southeast Asian J Trop Med Public Health. 2003 Mar;34(1):37-42.

234. Postma NS, Mommers EC, Eling WM, Zuidema J. Oxidative stress in malaria; implications for prevention and therapy. Pharm World Sci. 1996 Aug;18(4):121-9.

235. Kakkilaya, BS. The Malaria Site. Malaria Risk in Africa. Available from: http://www.malariasite.com/malaria/ artemisinin.htm. Accessed 2006 Aug 26.

236. Definition of Artemisinin. From MedicineNet.com. Available from: http://www.medterms.com/script/main/ art.asp?article key=24010. Accessed 2006 Aug 10.

237. Willcox M, Bodeker G, Bourdy G et al. Artemesia annua as a traditional herbal antimalarial. In: Traditional Medicinal Plants and Malaria. Eds. M. Willcox, G. Bodeker, P. Rasoanaivo. New York: CRC Press, 2004;p.52.

238. Wilairatana P, Looaresuwan S. The clinical use of artemisinin and its derivatives in the treatment of malaria. In Artemesia, Wright, CW, Ed. Taylor & Francis, London. 2002;p.298-299.

239. Lee J, Zhou HJ, Wu XH. Dihydroartemisinin downregulates vascular endothelial growth factor expression and

induces apoptosis in chronic myeloid leukemia K562 cells. Cancer Chemother Pharmacol. 2006;57:213-20. [Epub 2005 Aug 2].

240. Chen HH, Zhou HJ, Wang WQ, Wu GD. Antimalarial dihydroartemisinin also inhibits angiogenesis. Cancer Chemother Pharmacol. 2004 May;53(5):423-32.

241. Burk O, Arnold KA, Nussler AK, Schaeffeler E, Efimova E, Avery BA, Avery MA, Fromm MF, Eichelbaum M. Antimalarial artemisinin drugs induce cytochrome P450 and MDR1 expression by activation of xenosensors pregnane X receptor and constitutive androstane receptor. Mol Pharmacol. 2005;67:1954-65. [Epub 2005 Mar 10].

242. Bapiro TE, Sayi J, Hasler JA, Jande M, Rimoy G, Masselle A, Masimirembwa CM. Artemisinin and thiabendazole are potent inhibitors of cytochrome P450 1A2 (CYP1A2) activity in humans. Eur J Clin Pharmacol. 2005;61:755-61. [Epub 2005 Oct 29].

243. Simonsson US, Jansson B, Hai TN, Huong DX, Tybring G, Ashton M. Artemisinin autoinduction is caused by involvement of cytochrome P450 2B6 but not 2C9. Clin Pharmacol Ther. 2003;74:32-43.

244. Svensson US, Ashton M. Identification of the human cytochrome P450 enzymes involved in the in vitro metabolism of artemisinin. Br J Clin Pharmacol. 1999;48:528-35.

245. Xiao SH, Yao JM, Utzinger J, Cai Y, Chollet J, Tanner M. Selection and reversal of Plasmodium berghei resistance in the mouse model following repeated high doses

of artemether. Parasitol Res. 2004;92:215-9. [Epub 2003 Dec 16].

246. Chen YD, Lin BY, Zhang JX. Study on inducing an artemisinin-resistant line of Plasmodium berghei. Zhongguo Ji Sheng Chong Xue Yu Ji Sheng Chong Bing Za Zhi. 2002;20:37-8. [Article in Chinese].

247. SW Lininger, AR Gaby, S Austin, DR Brown, JV Wright, A Duncan. The Natural Pharmacy. 2nd edition. Rocklin CA; Prima Publishing, 1999;p.470-471.

248. Brewer TG, Grate SJ, Peggins JO, Weina PJ, Petras JM, Levine BS, Heiffer MH, Schuster BG. Fatal neurotoxicity of arteether and artemether. Am J Trop Med Hyg. 1994 Sept;51(3):251-9.

249. Li QG, Mog SR, Si YZ, Kyle DE, Gettayacamin M, Milhous WK. Neurotoxicity and efficacy of arteether related to its exposure times and exposure levels in rodents. Am J Trop Med Hyg. 2002 May;66(5):516-25.

250. Li QG, Brueckner RP, Peggins JO, Trotman KM, Brewer TG. Arteether toxicokinetics and pharmacokinetics in rats after 25 mg/kg/day single and multiple doses. Eur J Drug Metab Pharmacokinet. 1999 Jul-Sept;24(3):213-23.

251. Nontprasert A, Pukrittayakamee S, Prakongpan S, Supanaranond W, Looareesuwan S, White NJ. Assessment of the neurotoxicity of oral dihydroartemisinin in mice. Trans R Soc Trop Med Hyg. 2002 Jan-Feb;96(1):99-101.

252. Toovey S. Safety of Artemisinin Antimalarials. Clinical Infectious Diseases. 2006;42:1214-1215.

253. Peys E, Vandenkerckhove J, Van Hemel J, Sas B. Intermediate-term toxicity of repeated orally administered doses of the anti-malarial beta-artemether in dogs. Exp Toxicol Pathol. 2006;57:299-304. [Epub 2005 Dec, 20].

254. Kager PA, Schultz MJ, Zijlstra EE, et al, Arteether administration in humans: preliminary studies of pharmacokinetics, safety, and tolerance. Transactions of the Royal Society of Tropical Medicine and Hygiene. 1994;88:53-54.

255. Toovey S. Safety of Artemisinin Antimalarials. Clinical Infectious Diseases. 2006;42:1214-1215.

256. Toovey S, Jamieson A. Audiometric changes associated with the treatment of uncomplicated falciparum malaria with co-artemeter. Trans R Soc Trop Med Hyg. 2004;98:261-267.

257. Toovey S. Effects of weight, age, and time on artemether-lumefantrine associated ototoxicity and evidence of irreversibility. Travel Med Infect Dis. 2006;4:71-76.

258. Adjei G. Clinical neurotoxicity of artemisinin drugs in malaria treatment. In: Program and abstracts of the 4th Multilateral Initiative on Malaria conference. 2005.

259. The use of artemisinin and its derivatives as anti-malarial drugs. WHO/MAL/98.1086. Malaria Unit, Division of Control of Tropical Diseases, WHO, Geneva. 1998.

260. Wilairatana P, Looaresuwan S. The clinical use of artemisinin and its derivatives in the treatment of malaria. In Artemesia, Wright, CW, Ed. Taylor & Francis,

London. 2002.

261. Hien TT, Turner G, Mai NTH. Neuropathological assessment of artemether-treated severe malaria. Lancet. 2003;362:295-296.

262. Fishwick L, Edwards G, Ward SA, McLean WG. Binding of dihydroartemisinin to differentiating neuroblastoma cells and rat cortical homogenate. NeuroToxicology. 1998;19:405-412.

263. Fishwick L, Edwards G, Ward SA, McLean WG. Morphological and immunocytochemical effects of dihydroartemisinin on differentiating NB2a neuroblastoma cells. NeuroToxicity. 1998;19;393-403.

264. Fishwick L, McLean WG, Edwards G, Ward SA. The toxicity of artemisinin and related compounds on neuronal and glial cells in culture. Chem. Biol. Interact.1995;96:263-271.

265. Smith SL, Fishwick L, McLean WG, Edwards G, Ward SA. Enhanced in vitro neurotoxicity of artemisinin derivatives in the presence of haemin. Biochem. Pharmacol. 1997;53:5-10.

266. Kakkilaya, BS. The Malaria Site. Malaria Risk in Africa. Available from: http://www.malariasite.com/malaria/artemisinin.htm. Accessed August 2, 2006.

267. Gordi T, Lepist EI. Artemisinin derivatives: toxic for laboratory animals, safe for humans? Toxicol Lett. 2004 Mar 1;147(2):99-107.

268. Gordi T, Lepist EI. Toxicol Lett. 2004 Aug 1;151(3):489-90, author reply 491-2. Acta Trop. 2002 May;82(2)175-81.

269. Clark RL, White TE, A Clode S, Gaunt I, Winstanley P, Ward SA. Developmental toxicity of artesunate and an artesunate combination in the rat and rabbit. Birth Defects Res B Dev Reprod Toxicol. 2004 Dec; 71(6):380-94.

270. Hutagalung R, Htoo H, Nwee P, Arunkamomkiri J, Zwang J, Car-rara VI, Ashley E, Singhasivanon P, White NJ, Nosten F. A case-control auditory evaluation of patients treated with artemether-lumefantrine. Am J Trop Med Hyg. 2006 Feb;74(2):211-4.

271. Xiao S, Tanner M, N'Goran EK, Utzinger J, Chollet J, Bergquist R, Chen M, Zheng J. Recent investigations of artemether, a novel agent for the prevention of schisto-somiasis japonica, mansoni and haematobia. Acta Trop. 2002 May;82(2):175-81.

272. Xiao S, Tanner M, N'Goran EK, Utzinger J, Chollet J, Bergquist R, Chen M, Zheng J. Recent investigations of artemether, a novel agent for the prevention of schisto-somiasis japonica, mansoni and haematobia. Acta Trop. 2002 May;82(2):175-81.

273. Hung le Q, de Vries PJ, Binh TQ, Giao PT, Nam NV, Holman R, Kager PA. Artesunate with mefloquine at various intervals for non-severe Plasmodium falciparum malaria. Am J Trop Med Hyg. 2004 Aug;71(2):160-6.

274. Tangpukdee N, Krudsood S, Thanachartwet W, Chalermrut K, Pengruksa C, Srivilairit S, Silachamroon U, Wilairatana P, Phong-tananant S, Kano S, Looareesuwan S. An open randomized clinical trial of Artekin vs artesunate-mefloquine in the treatment of acute uncomplicated falciparum malaria. Southeast Asian

J Trop Med Public Health. 2005 Sept;36(5):1085-91.

275. Peys E, Vandenkerckhove J, Van Hemel J, Sas B. Intermediate-term toxicity of repeated orally administered doses of the anti-malarial beta-artemether in dogs. Exp Toxicol Pathol. 2006 Mar;57(4):299-304. [Epub 2005 Dec 20].

276. Dayan AD. Neurotoxicity and artemisinin compounds do the observations in animals justify limitation of clinical use? Med Trop (Mars). 1998;58(3 Suppl):32-7.

277. Fishwick J, Edwards G, Ward SA, McLean WG. Morphological and immunocytochemical effects of dihydroartemisinin on differentiating NB2a neuroblastoma cells. Neurotoxicology. 1998;19:393-403.

278. Smith SL, Sadler CJ, Dodd CC, Edwards G, Ward SA, Park BK, McLean WG. The role of glutathione in the neurotoxicity of artemisinin derivatives in vitro. Biochem Pharmacol. 2001 Feb 15;61(4):409-16.

279. Panossian LA, Garga NI, Pelletier D. Toxic brainstem encephalopathy after artemisinin treatment for breast cancer. Ann. Neurol 2005;56;812-813.

280. Gordi T, Xie R, Huong NV, Huong DX, Karlsson MO, Ashton M. A semiphysiological pharmacokinetic model for artemisinin in healthy subjects incorporating autoinduction of metabolism and saturable first-pass hepatic extraction. Br J Clin Pharmacol. 2005 Feb;59(2):189-98.

281. Van Agtmael MA, Eggelte TA and CJ van Boxtel. Artmisinin drugs in the treatment of malaria: from medicinal herb to registered medication. Trends Pharmacol. Sci. 1999;20:199-205. Available from:

http://www.malariasite.com/malaria/ artemisinin.htm. Accessed 2006 Aug 7.

282. Kakkilaya BS. Malaria Risk In Africa. From the Malaria Site, All About Malaria. Available from: http://www. malariasite.com/malaria/artemisinin.htm. Accessed 2006 Aug 12.

283. Kakkilaya BS. Malaria Risk In Africa. From the Malaria Site, All About Malaria. Available from: http://www. malariasite.com/malaria/artemisinin.htm. Accessed 2006 Aug 13.

284. Zhang Q, Zhang Y. Lyme disease and modern Chinese medicine. Sino-Med Reseach Institute, New York, NY. 2006;p.34-35 and see treatment flow chart.

285. Zhang Q, Zhang Y. Lyme disease and modern Chinese medicine. Sino-Med Reseach Institute, New York, NY. 2006;p.34-35,42-43.

286. Phillips-Howard P. Regulation of the quality and use of artemesinin and its derivatives. In Artemesia, Wright, CW, Ed. Taylor & Francis, London. 2002;p.319-320.

287. Kakkilaya BS. Malaria Risk In Africa. From the Malaria Site, All About Malaria. [Monograph on the Internet]. Available from: http://www.malariasite.com/malaria/ artemisinin.htm. Accessed 2006 Aug 13.

288. Phillips-Howard P. Regulation of the quality and use of artemesinin and its derivatives. In Artemesia, Wright, CW, Ed. Taylor & Francis, London. 2002;p.319-320.

289. Phillips-Howard P. Regulation of the quality and use of artemesinin and its derivatives. In Artemesia, Wright, CW, Ed. Taylor & Francis, London. 2002;p.319-320.

290. Kakkilaya BS. Malaria Risk In Africa. From the Malaria Site, All About Malaria. [Monograph on the Internet]. Available from: http://www.malariasite.com/malaria/ artemisinin.htm. Accessed Aug 13, 2006.260. Le NH, Na-Bangchang K, Le TD, Thrinh KA, Karbwang J. Phamacokinetics of a single oral dose of dihydroartemisinin in Vietnamese healthy volunteers. Southeast Asian J Trop Med Public Health. 1999;30:11-6.

291. Le NH, Na-Bangchang K, Le TD, Thrinh KA, Karbwang J. Phamacokinetics of a single oral dose of dihydroartemisinin in Vietnamese healthy volunteers. Southeast Asian J Trop Med Public Health. 1999 Mar;30(1):11-6.

292. Sabine Bork, Naoaki Yokoyama, Yuzuru Ikehara, Sanjay Kumar, Chihiro Sugimoto, and Ikuo Igarashi. Growth-Inhibitory Effect of Heparin on Babesia Parasites. In: Antimicrobial Agents and Chemotherapy. Jan. 2004;48:1:236–241.

293. Sabine Bork, Naoaki Yokoyama, Yuzuru Ikehara, Sanjay Kumar, Chihiro Sugimoto, and Ikuo Igarashi. ANTIMI-CROBIAL AGENTS AND CHEMOTHERAPY, Jan. 2004;p.236-241;Vol. 48, No. 1. Growth-Inhibitory Effect of Heparin on Babesia Parasites.

294. CF Lacy, LL Armstrong, MP Goldman, LL Lance. Drug Information Handbook. 14th edition. Hudson, Ohio: Lexi-Comp; 2006. p. 1366-1367.

295. Falagas ME, Klempner MS. Babesiosis in patients with AIDS: a chronic infection presenting as fever of unknown origin. Clin Infect Dis. 1996 May;22(5):809-12. Available from: http://www.rxlist.com/cgi/gener-

ic2/clindam_cp.htm.

296. From Clindamycin: Medline Plus. [Monograph on the Internet]. Available from: http://www.nlm.nih.gov/medlineplus/druginfo/medmaster/a682399.html.

297. From RXList. [Monograph on the Internet]. Available from: http://www.rxlist.com/cgi/generic2/clindam_cp.htm.

298. From Clindamycin: Medline Plus. [Monograph on the Internet]. Available from: http://www.nlm.nih.gov/medlineplus/druginfo/medmaster/a682399.html.

299. Mermin J, Ekwaru JP, Liechty CA, Were W, Downing R, Ransom R, Weidle P, Lule J, Coutinho A, Solberg P. Effect of co-trimoxazole prophylaxis, antiretroviral therapy, and insecticide-treated bednets on the frequency of malaria in HIV-1-infected adults in Uganda: a prospective cohort study. Lancet. 2006 Apr 15;367(9518):1256-61.

300. Sowunmi A, Gbotosho GO, Fateye BA, Adedeji AA. Predictors of the failure of treatment with trimethoprim-sulfamethoxazole in children with uncomplicated, Plasmodium falciparum malaria. Ann Trop Med Parasitol. 2006 Apr;100(3):205-11.

301. Thera MA, Sehdev PS, Coulibaly D, Traore K, Garba MN, Cissoko Y, Kone A, Guindo A, Dicko A, Beavogui AH, Djimde AA, Lyke KE, Diallo DA, Doumbo OK, Plowe CV. Impact of trimethoprim-sulfamethoxazole prophylaxis on falciparum malaria infection and disease. J Infect Dis. 2005 Nov 15;192(10):1823-9. Epub 2005 Oct 13.

302. Hamel MJ, Holtz T, Mkandala C, Kaimila N, Chizani N, Bloland P, Kublin J, Kazembe P, Steketee R. Efficacy of

trimethoprim-sulfamethoxazole compared with sulfa-doxine-pyrimethamine plus erythromycin for the treatment of uncomplicated malaria in children with integrated management of childhood illness dual classifications of malaria and pneumonia. Am J Trop Med Hyg. 2005 Sep;73(3):609-15.

303. Chong CR, Sullivan DJ Jr. Inhibition of heme crystal growth by antimalarials and other compounds: implications for drug discovery. Biochem Pharmacol. 2003 Dec 1;66(11):2201-12.

304. From: Medline Plus: Doxycycline. [Monograph on the Internet]. Available from: http://www.nlm.nih.gov/medlineplus/druginfo/uspdi/500643.html.

305. Van Heerden J, Reyers F, Stewart CG. Treatment and thrombocyte levels in experimentally induced canine ehrlichiosis and canine babesiosis. Onderstepoort J Vet Res. 1983 Dec;50(4):267-70.

306. Menichetti F, Bindi ML, Tascini C, Urbani L, Biancofiore G, Doria R, Esposito M, Mozzo R, Catalano G, Filipponi F. Fever, mental impairment, acute anemia, and renal failure in patient undergoing orthotopic liver transplantation: posttransplantation malaria. Liver Transpl. 2006 Apr;12(4):674-6.

307. Miller RS, Wongsrichanalai C, Buathong N, McDaniel P, Walsh DS, Knirsch C, Ohrt C. Effective treatment of uncomplicated Plasmodium falciparum malaria with azithromycin-quinine combinations: a randomized, dose-ranging study. Am J Trop Med Hyg. 2006 Mar;74(3):401-6.

308. Falagas ME, Klempner MS. Babesiosis in patients with AIDS: a chronic infection presenting as fever of unknown origin. Clin Infect Dis. 1996 May;22(5):809-12.

309. Leggat PA. Trends in antimalarial prescriptions in Australia from 1998 to 2002. J Travel Med. 2005 Nov-Dec;12(6):338-42.

310. Schwartz E, Regev-Yochay G. Primaquine as prophylaxis for malaria for nonimmune travelers: A comparison with mefloquine and doxycycline. Clin Infect Dis. 1999 Dec;29(6):1502-6.

311. From: Medline Plus: Doxycycline. [Monograph on the Internet]. Available from: http://www.nlm.nih.gov/medlineplus/druginfo/uspdi/500643.htm.

312. CF Lacy, LL Armstrong, MP Goldman, LL Lance. Drug Information Handbook. 14th edition. Hudson, Ohio: Lexi-Comp; 2006. p.795-796.

313. Romanelli F, Smith KM, Hoven AD. Chloroquine and hydroxychloroquine as inhibitors of human immunodeficiency virus (HIV-1) activity. Curr Pharm Des. 2004;10(21):2643-8.

314. Warhurst DC, Steele JC, Adagu IS, Craig JC, Cullander C. Hydroxychloroquine is much less active than chloroquine against chloroquine-resistant Plasmodium falciparum, in agreement with its physicochemical properties. J Antimicrob Chemother. 2003 Aug;52(2):188-93. Epub 2003 Jul 1.

315. From: Medline Plus: Drugs and Supplements. "Hydroxychloroquine". [Monograph on the Internet].

Available from: http://www.nlm.nih.gov/medlineplus/ druginfo/medmaster/a601240.html.

316. From: Sanofi-Synthelabo: Prescribing Information. [Monograph on the Internet]. Available from: http://products.sanofiaventis.us/plaquenil/plaquenil.html.

317. Koranda FC. Antimalarials. J Am Acad Dermatol. 1981 Jun;4(6):650-5.

318. Fardet L, Revuz J. [Synthetic antimalarials]. Ann Dermatol Venereol. 2005 Aug-Sep;132(8-9 Pt 1):665-74.

319. Weisinger HS, Pesudovs K, Collin HB. Management of patients undergoing hydroxychloroquine (Plaquenil) therapy. Clin Exp Optom. 2000 Jan;83(1):32-36.

320. Wei LC, Chen SN, Ho CL, Kuo YH, Ho JD. Progression of hydroxychloroquine retinopathy after discontinuation of therapy: case report. Chang Gung Med J. 2001 May;24(5):329-34.

321. Rebholz CE, Michel AJ, Maselli DA Dr, Saipphudin K Dr, Wyss K Dr. Frequency of malaria and glucose-6-phosphate dehydrogenase deficiency in Tajikistan. Malar J. 2006 Jun 16;5(1):51 [Epub ahead of print].

322. Ferraro V, Mantoux F, Denis K, Lay-Macagno MA, Ortonne JP, Lacour JP. Hallucinations during treatment with hydrochloroquine. Ann Dermatol Venereol. 2004 May;131(5):471-3. [Article in French].

323. Koren G. Antimalarial drugs for rheumatoid disease during pregnancy. Can Fam Physician. 1999 Dec;45:2869-70.

324. Levy M, Buskila D, Gladman DD, Urowitz MB, Koren G. Pregnancy outcome following first trimester exposure to chloroquine. Am J Perinatol. 1991 May;8 (3):174-8.

325. Penzhorn BL, Schoeman T, Jacobson LS. Feline babesiosis in South Africa: a review. Ann N Y Acad Sci. 2004 Oct;1026:183-6.

326. Penzhorn BL, Lewis BD, Lopez-Rebollar LM, Swan GE. Screening of five drugs for efficacy against Babesia felis in experimentally infected cats. J S Afr Vet Assoc. 2000 Mar;71(1):53-7.

327. Egan TJ. Chloroquine and primaquine: combining old drugs as a new weapon against falciparum malaria? Trends Parasitol. 2006 Jun;22(6):235-7. Epub 2006 Apr 3.

328. Munoz J, Velasco M, Alonso D, Valls ME, Corachan M, Gascon J. How much primaquine is needed to eradicate Plasmodium vivax hypnozoites? Enferm Infecc Microbiol Clin. 2006 Jan;24(1):29-30. [Article in Spanish].

329. Schwartz E. Regev-Yochay G. Primaquine as prophylaxis for malaria for nonimmune travelers: A comparison with mefloquine and doxycycline. Clin Infect Dis. 1999 Dec;29(6):1502-6.

330. Kitchen LW, Vaughn DW, Skillman DR. Role of US military research programs in the development of US food and drug administration-approved antimaleria drugs. Reviews of anti-infective agents. 2006;43:67-71.

331. Greenburg, S. G6PD Deficiency. [Monograph on the

Internet]. Available from: http://www.utoronto.ca/ kids/G6PD.htm.

332. From: University of Virginia Health System. Hematology and Blood Disorders. What is G6PD Deficiency? [Monograph on the Internet]. Available from: http://www.healthsystem.virginia.edu/ uva-health/adult_blood/glucose.cfm.

333. Potgieter FT. Chemotherapy of Babesia felis infection: efficacy of certain drugs. J S Afr Vet Assoc. 1981 Dec;52(4):289-93.

334. CF Lacy, LL Armstrong, MP Goldman, LL Lance. Drug Information Handbook. 14th edition. Hudso, Ohio: Lexi-Comp; 2006. p. 1315-1316.

335. Cuong BT, Binh VQ, Dai B, Duy DN, Lovell CM, Rieckmann KH, Edstein MD. Does gender, food or grapefruit juice alter the pharmacokinetics of primaquine in healthy subjects? Br J Clin Pharmacol. 2006 Jun;61(6):682-9.

336. Shoemaker RC, Hudnell HK, House DE, Van Kempen A, Pakes GE; COL40155 Study Team. Atovaquone plus cholestyramine in patients coinfected with Babesia microti and Borrelia burgdorferi refractory to other treatment. Available from http://www.Pubmed.org.

337. Clark IA. Does endotoxin cause both the disease and parasite death in acute malaria and babasiosis? Lancet. 1978;2:75-7.

338. Commins MA, Goodger BV, Waltisbuhl DJ, Wright IG. Babesia bovis: studies of parameters influencing microvascular stasis of infected erythrocytes. Res Vet

Sci. 1988 Mar;44(2):226-8.

339. Naik RS, Krishnegowda G, Gowda DC. Glucosamine inhibits inosital acylation of the glycosylphosphatidyli-nositol anchors in itraerythrocytic Plasmodium falci-parum. J Biol Chem. 2003;278:2036-42.

340. Dupouy-Camet J. New drugs for the treatment of human parasitic protozoa. [Article in French]. Parassitologia. 2004 Jun;46(1-2):81-4.

341. Alinia. Package Insert. Accessed 2006 September 10. Available from: http://www.romark.com.

342. Alinia. Package Insert. Accessed 2006 September 10. Available from: http://www.romark.com.

343. Marley SE, Eberhard ML, Steurer FJ, Ellis WL, McGreevy PB, Ruebush TK 2nd. Evaluation of selected antiprotozoal drugs in the Babesia microti-hamster model. Antimicrob Agents Chemother. 1997 Jan;41(1):91-4.

344. McCarthy, JS. Malaria Chemoprophylaxis in War and Peace. [Editorial]. MJA vol. 182 No. 4, 2005 Feb. 21. Available from: http://www.mja.com.au/public/issues/182_04_210205/mcc10925_fm.pdf.

345. Thomas, MJG. Occasional Newsletter from the Blood Care Foundation. 2003 Dec. 3. www.bloodcare.org.uk/pdfs/Newsletter%20No%2021.pdf Accessed 2006 Sept 1.

346. McCarthy, JS. Malaria Chemoprophylaxis in War and Peace. [Editorial]. MJA vol. 182 No. 4, 2005 Feb. 21. Available from: http://www.mja.com.au/public/issues/182_04_210205/mcc10925_fm.pdf.

347. From: Health24.com. Travel Health: About Travel Health. Malaria. [Monograph on the Internet]. Available from: http://health.mweb.co.za/medical/Condition_centres/777-792-824-1855,11956.asp.

348. Thomas, MJG. Occasional Newsletter from the Blood Care Foundation. 2003 Dec. 3. www.bloodcare.org.uk/pdfs/Newsletter%20No%2021.pdf Accessed 2006 Sept 1.

349. Douglas S. Walsh, Sornchai Looareesuwan, Polrat Wilairatana, D. Gray Heppner, Jr., Douglas B. Tang, Thomas G. Brewer, Watcharee Chokejindachai, Parnpen Viriyavejakul, Dennis E. Kyle, Wilbur K. Milhous, Brian G. Schuster, John Horton, David J. Braitman, and Ralf P. Brueckner Randomized Dose-Ranging Study of the Safety and Efficacy of WR 238605 (Tafenoquine) in the Prevention of Relapse of Plasmodium vivax Malaria in Thailand. The Journal of Infectious Diseases, Vol. 180. 1999; p.1282–1287.

350. Walsh DS, Eamsila C, Sasiprapha T, Sangkharomya S, Khaewsathien P, Supakalin P, Tang DB, Jarasrumgsichol P, Cherdchu C, Edstein MD, Rieckmann KH, Brewer TG. Efficacy of monthly tafenoquine for prophylaxis of Plasmodium vivax and multidrug-resistant P. falciparum malaria. J Infect Dis. 2004 Oct 15;190(8):1456-63. Epub 2004 Sep 20.

351. Nasveld P, Kitchener S. Treatment of acute vivax malaria with tafenoquine. Trans R Soc Trop Med Hyg. 2005 Jan;99(1):2-5.

352. Michael D. Edstein, David A. Kocisko, Thomas G. Brewer, Douglas S. Walsh, Chirapa Eamsila, & Bruce

G. Charles. Population pharmacokinetics of the new antimalarial agent tafenoquine in Thai soldiers. British Journal of Clinical Pharmacology. 2001 Dec. Vol. 52;p.663.

353. Edstein MD, Nasveld PE, Kocisko DA, Kitchener SJ, Gatton ML, Rieckmann KH. Gender differences in gastrointestinal disturbances and plasma concentrations of tafenoquine in healthy volunteers after tafenoquine administration for post-exposure vivax malaria prophylaxis. Trans R Soc Trop Med Hyg. 2006 Jun 29; [Epub ahead of print].

354. Milhous W. Development of new drugs for chemoprophylaxis of malaria. Bull Soc Pathol Exot. 2001 Jul;94(2 Pt 2):149-51.

355. Shanks GD, Edstein MD. Modern malaria chemoprophylaxis. Drugs. 2005;65(15):2091-110.

356. Walsh DS, Wilairatana P, Tang DB, Heppner DG Jr, Brewer TG, Krudsood S, Silachamroon U, Phumratanaprapin W, Siriyanonda D, Looareesuwan S. Randomized trial of 3-dose regimens of tafenoquine (WR238605) versus low-dose primaquine for preventing Plasmodium vivax malaria relapse. Clin Infect Dis. 2004 Oct 15;39(8):1095-103. Epub 2004 Sep 24.

357. Thomas, MJG. Occasional Newsletter from the Blood Care Foundation. 2003 Dec. 3. www.bloodcare.org.uk/pdfs/Newsletter%20No% 2021.pdf Accessed 2006 Sept 1.

358. Hale BR, Owusu-Agyei S, Fryauff DJ, Koram KA, Adjuik M, Oduro AR, Prescott WR, Baird JK, Nkrumah

F, Ritchie TL, Franke ED, Binka FN, Horton J, Hoffman SL. A randomized, double-blind, placebo-controlled, dose-ranging trial of tafenoquine for weekly prophylaxis against Plasmodium falciparum. Clin Infect Dis. 2003 Mar 1;36(5):541-9. [Epub. 2003 Feb 14].

359. Puri SK, Dutta GP. Blood schizontocidal activity of WR 238605 (Tafenoquine) against Plasmodium cynomolgi and Plasmodium fragile infections in rhesus monkeys. Acta Trop. 2003 Apr;86(1):35-40.

360. Edstein MD, Kocisko DA, Walsh DS, Eamsila C, Charles BG, Rieckmann KH. Plasma concentrations of tafenoquine, a new long-acting antimalarial agent, in thai soldiers receiving monthly prophylaxis. Clin Infect Dis. 2003 Dec 15;37(12):1654-8. Epub 2003 Nov 20.

361. Ramharter M, Noedl H, Thimasarn K, Wiedermann G, Wernsdorfer G, Wernsdorfer WH. In vitro activity of tafenoquine alone and in combination with artemisinin against Plasmodium falciparum. Am J Trop Med Hyg. 2002 Jul;67(1):39-43.

362. Ohrt C, Willingmyre GD, Lee P, Knirsch C, Milhous W. Assessment of azithromycin in combination with other antimalarial drugs against Plasmodium falciparum in vitro. Antimicrob Agents Chemother. 2002 Aug;46;(8):2518-24.

363. Subeki, Nomura S, Matsuura H, Yamasaki M, Yamato O, Maede Y, Katakura K, Suzuki M, Trimurningsih, Chairul, Yoshihara T. Anti-babesial activity of some central kalimantan plant extracts and active oligostilbenoids from Shorea balangeran. Planta Med. 2005 May;71(5):420-3.

364. Fox LM, Wingerter S, Ahmed A, Arnold A, Chou J, Rhein L, Levy O. Neonatal babesiosis: case report and review of the literature. Pediatr Infect Dis J. 2006 Feb;25(2):169-73.

365. Baspinar O, Bayraktaroglu Z, Karsligil T, Bayram A, Coskun Y. A rare cause of anemia and thrombocytopenia in a newborn: congenital malaria. Turk J Pediatr. Department of Pediatrics, Gaziantep University Faculty of Medicine, Gaziantep, Turkey. 2006 Jan-Mar;48(1):63-5.

366. Zenz W, Trop M, Kollaritsch H, Reinthaler F. Congenital malaria due to Plasmodium falciparum and Plasmodium malariae. Wien Klin Wochenschr. 2000 May 19;112(10):459-61. [Article in German]. Comment in: Wien Klin Wochenschr. 2000 May 19;112(10):421-2.

367. Dummond R, Ticks and what you can do about them. Wilderness Press;Berkeley, CA: 2004. p.59-69.

368. Westport Westin Health District. Available at: http://www. wwhd.org.

Other Books By Dr. Schaller

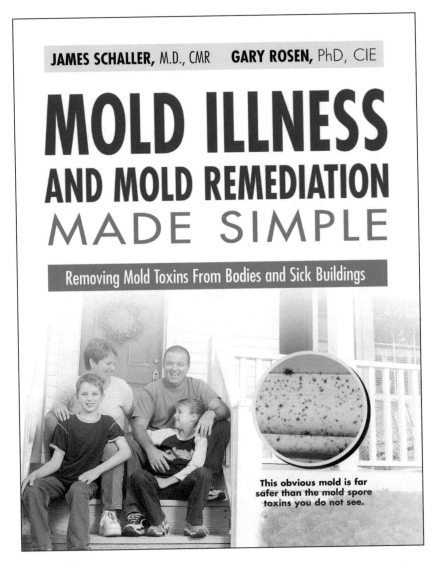

JAMES SCHALLER, M.D., CMR   **GARY ROSEN,** PhD, CIE

MOLD ILLNESS
AND MOLD REMEDIATION
MADE SIMPLE

Removing Mold Toxins From Bodies and Sick Buildings

This obvious mold is far safer than the mold spore toxins you do not see.

Dr. Schaller is both a certified mold investigator and a certified mold remediator. He has authored or co-authored three books on indoor mold biotoxins. If you have been exposed to mold that can be seen or smelled, you should consider buying this book. It is the only book available which offers both **profoundly** clear writing and up-to-date useful information on mold illnesses and mold remediation. It is written with pictures and amusing comics in a manner that allows you to understand indoor mold rapidly. Further, if you struggle with reading books with small print or that require extended periods of concentration, this book is the perfect solution.

* * * * *

This book is available as an E-book from www.HopeAcademic.com. A soft-cover copy is also available from Amazon.com.

Other Books By Dr. Schaller

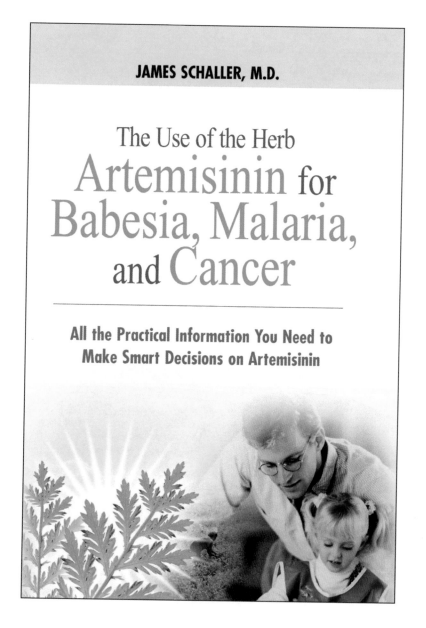

JAMES SCHALLER, M.D.

The Use of the Herb
Artemisinin for Babesia, Malaria, and Cancer

All the Practical Information You Need to Make Smart Decisions on Artemisinin

This is the first book in the English language which discusses clearly and thoroughly practical information distilled from the available research. This unique herb is the first line treatment for malaria worldwide, and some patients report it has helped them with Babesia infections. It also appears to hold promise for oncology in the treatment of select cancers.

* * * * *

This book is available as an E-book from www.HopeAcademic.com. A soft-cover copy is also available from Amazon.com.

Other Books By Dr. Schaller

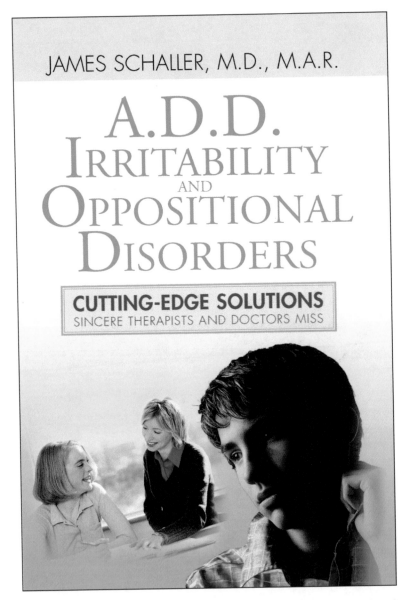

Dr. Schaller routinely discovers missed causes of emotional and behavior problems in small children and adolescents. His typical child patient has already been evaluated by many smart child and adolescent psychiatrists, child psychologists and pediatricians. In this highly unique and highly practical book, Dr. Schaller offers both causes and solutions to parents who want their child to function better and be as happy as possible.

* * * * *

This book is available as an E-book from www.HopeAcademic.com. A soft-cover copy is also available from Amazon.com.

Other Books By Dr. Schaller

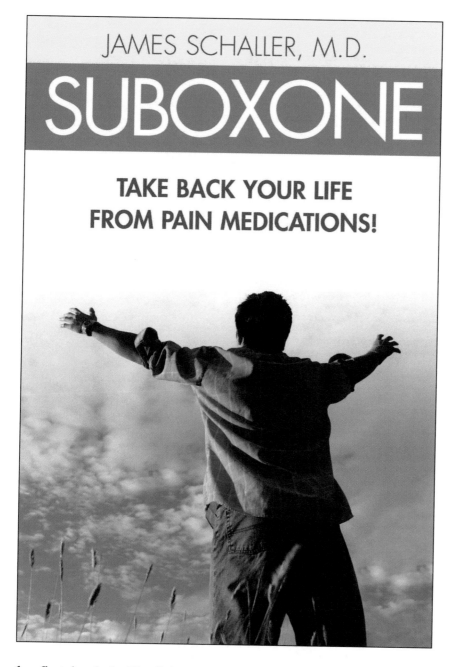

JAMES SCHALLER, M.D.

SUBOXONE

TAKE BACK YOUR LIFE FROM PAIN MEDICATIONS!

This is the first book in English written for patients about Suboxone. It offers exciting information about this excellent pain medication, which also is the most important new treatment for narcotic addiction in the last thirty years.

* * * * *

This book is available as an E-book from www.HopeAcademic.com. A soft-cover copy is also available from Amazon.com.

Other Books By Dr. Schaller

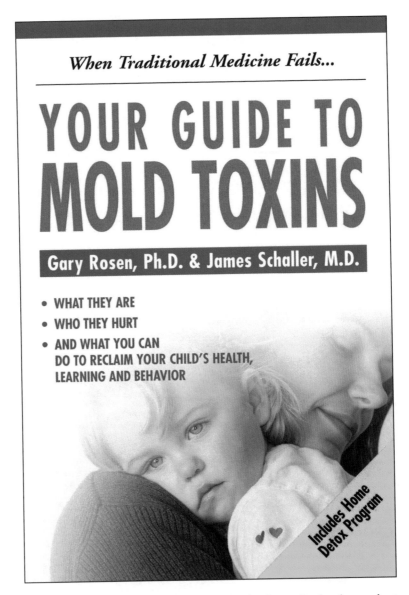

When Traditional Medicine Fails...

YOUR GUIDE TO MOLD TOXINS

Gary Rosen, Ph.D. & James Schaller, M.D.

- WHAT THEY ARE
- WHO THEY HURT
- AND WHAT YOU CAN DO TO RECLAIM YOUR CHILD'S HEALTH, LEARNING AND BEHAVIOR

Includes Home Detox Program

In 2004, the EPA warned physicians to be on the lookout for both respiratory and neurological symptoms from mold contaminated schools and homes. The latest medical science shows 1 in 4 children are sensitive to low levels of mold toxins. Is your child one of these? Now a "Top Gun" physician and medical innovator teams up with an accomplished scientist and master builder to clearly explain how even small amounts of hidden indoor mold can produce biotoxins which can subtly impact youth behavior, emotions, health and learning.   * * * * *

This book is available as an E-book from www.HopeAcademic.com. A soft-cover copy is also available from Amazon.com.

Dr. Schaller has been published in the following Journals and Newspapers:

Journal of the American Medical Association

Journal of Clinical Neuroscience

Medscape (Academic Journal of WebMD)

Journal of the American Society of Child and Adolescent Psychiatry

American Journal of Psychiatry

European Journal of Child and Adolescent Psychiatry

Compounding Pharmaceuticals: Triad

Fleming Revell Press (Four Languages)

Internal Medicine News

Family Practice News

Spire Mass Market Books

Internet Journal of Family Medicine

Child and Adolescent Psychiatry Drug Alerts

Clinical Psychiatry News

Psychiatric Drug Alerts

Townsend Journal

OB/GYN News

AMA News

Currents

To Contact Dr. Schaller:

Tampa:
Office Suites Plus
7320 E. Fletcher Ave.
Tampa, FL 33637
USA
Phone: 813-909-8009

Naples:
Community Bank Towers
Newgate Center, Suite 305
5150 Tamiami Trail N
Naples, FL 34103
USA
Phone: 239-263-0133